Anatomy, Modeling and Biomaterial Fabrication for Dental and Maxillofacial Applications

Authored by

Andy H. Choi and Besim Ben-Nissan

Advanced Tissue Regeneration & Drug Delivery Group, School of Life Science, Faculty of Science, University of Technology Sydney, Australia

Anatomy, Modeling and Biomaterial Fabrication for Dental and Maxillofacial Applications

Authors: Andy H. Choi and Besim Ben-Nissan

ISBN (Online): 978-1-68108-691-0

ISBN (Print): 978-1-68108-692-7

General:

1. Any dispute or claim arising out of or in connection with this License Agreement or the Work (including non-contractual disputes or claims) will be governed by and construed in accordance with the laws of the U.A.E. as applied in the Emirate of Dubai. Each party agrees that the courts of the Emirate of Dubai shall have exclusive jurisdiction to settle any dispute or claim arising out of or in connection with this License Agreement or the Work (including non-contractual disputes or claims).
2. Your rights under this License Agreement will automatically terminate without notice and without the need for a court order if at any point you breach any terms of this License Agreement. In no event will any delay or failure by Bentham Science Publishers in enforcing your compliance with this License Agreement constitute a waiver of any of its rights.
3. You acknowledge that you have read this License Agreement, and agree to be bound by its terms and conditions. To the extent that any other terms and conditions presented on any website of Bentham Science Publishers conflict with, or are inconsistent with, the terms and conditions set out in this License Agreement, you acknowledge that the terms and conditions set out in this License Agreement shall prevail.

Bentham Science Publishers Ltd.
Executive Suite Y - 2
PO Box 7917, Saif Zone
Sharjah, U.A.E.
Email: subscriptions@benthamscience.org

**BENTHAM
SCIENCE**

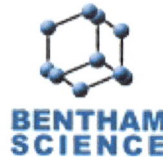

CONTENTS

FOREWORD

The use of biomaterials has been a mainstay in oral and maxillofacial applications. In recent years, better understanding of biological and biomolecular responses to implant materials as well as advances in biomaterial engineering, have led to the development of novel biomaterials which incorporate various aspects of tissue engineering, regenerative medicine, nanotechnology, surface functionalization and composite systems. A key consideration in biomaterial engineering is biocompatibility, which is the ability for the implant biomaterial to illicit an appropriate host tissue response whilst avoiding and preventing undesirable effects. This consideration is highly specific to the intended function and site where the implant is being used. As such, keen appreciation of the physiology and anatomy of the implant site will be required during material selection and design.

Amongst various metallic biomaterials, use of titanium and its alloys (Ti-6Al-4V) is one of the most widespread for oral and maxillofacial applications. Since its first use, titanium implants have the longest traceable record in clinical practice, receiving a success rate as high as 99 % for 15 years. Good biocompatibility, favorable tissue response, adequate strength and corrosion resistance are some of the key attributes which make it an excellent choice as a biomaterial worldwide. An important property to titanium's good biocompatibility is its ability to form an oxide layer almost spontaneously when exposed to air, and it is this oxide layer which not only passivates the bulk metal, but more importantly induces apatite formation (the main inorganic component of natural bone) when implanted. However, the use of titanium implants is not without certain issues. Incomplete osteointegration can still occur where there is insufficient contact between the metal and host bone. Methods to address these issues include surface modifications (sand blasting, acid etching, plasma coating to name a few) to increase surface roughness, oxide layer and bioactivity.

Ceramics have been used as biomaterials for oral and maxillofacial applications due to their properties of good bioactivity, high hardness and wear resistance. Bioceramics can be categorized based on the biological response when they are implanted: bioinert or bioactive. Bioinert medical materials generally do not result in any host tissue response, and remain in the implant site without osteointegration. Bioactive medical materials provide a conducive environment which interacts and changes with its implanted environment. With bioceramics, bioactivity is commonly associated with osteoconductivity, whereby the biomaterial functions to guide and facilitate bone attachment and in-growth. However, bioceramics are typically brittle in nature, and cannot be used alone in high load-bearing applications. Some of the common bioceramics are apatites, calcium phosphates and bioglass.

Nanotechnology refers to the manipulation, synthesis and fabrication of materials at the nanometer-scale. It has been widely regarded as a tool which will enable the engineering of next generation biomaterials. Applications of nanomaterials in oral and maxillofacial health is becoming increasingly common due to numerous advantages, which can be realized through engineering at the nanometer-scale. Nanostructured materials display physical properties which are distinctly different from the same material at the micrometer-scale. At the cellular level, nanoengineered features have been shown to elicit specific biological responses. Even recent efforts at elucidating of cell-cell, cell-matrix interactions have been focused on nanometer-scale material manipulation, targeting specific up-regulation and signaling pathways. Indeed, nanostructured titanium implants have shown to promote osteoblast adhesion, spreading and proliferation. Ligand specific signaling through nanoscale Arg-Gl--Asp (RGD) functionalization on titanium surfaces have also shown to improve osteointegration. Nanosized calcium phosphate coatings on implant surfaces through sol-gel transformation have also reported to improve implant mineralization. Thus, materials previously regarded as inadequate for osteointegration may be considered once more due to nanosurface functionalization.

Nanomaterials offer the advantage of very high surface to volume ratio, and are relevant as carriers for targeted and controlled delivery of growth factors, drugs and other therapeutic substances. They can enable the realization of tissue regeneration, where diseases can be treated by injecting these nanomaterials to deliver the therapy in a spatially and temporally controlled manner. A large portion of failures in oral and maxillofacial treatment and complications is due to recurrent microbial infection, leading to implant failure. Incorporation of silver nanoparticles has been shown to improve the antimicrobial properties, significantly. Furthermore, smaller-sized silver nanoparticles have been associated with greater efficacy, owing to their increased surface to volume ratio and ability to disrupt bacteria membrane, effectively.

In conclusion, biomaterials play a pervasive and integral role in oral and maxillofacial applications. Through greater understanding of physiology and biomolecular processes, better considerations can be made to the selection, design and development of biomaterials. Owing to the diverse function that each tissue plays, various metals and ceramics have been used for specific oral and maxillofacial applications. These materials can also be incorporated as composites to overcome shortcomings of an individual material. Advances in engineering techniques, in particularly nanotechnology, have opened up a myriad of possibilities which promise to revolutionize the way biomaterials are made and improve biomedical outcomes significantly. Future research endeavors should continue elucidating the mechanism of osteointegration, uncover specific implant-tissue responses and their associated internal mechanism, thereby improving on our model of biomaterial engineering.

Eng San Thian
Ph.D. (Cambridge)
Department of Mechanical Engineering
National University of Singapore
Singapore

PREFACE

This book is divided into four major sections. The first section provides basic insights into human anatomy including the structure of bone and the functional anatomy of the skull. The next two sections focus on the applications of mathematical and computerized modeling methodology in dentistry as well as in oral and maxillofacial surgery, not only at a research level but also at a clinical level. Mathematical models and experimental studies are two distinct approaches that can be used to further our understanding of the stress and strain environment in mammalian jaw. Despite the fact that accuracy as well as the possibility (to a certain extent) of characterizing the biomechanical behavior of the mandible are offered by experimental studies, mathematical approaches provide unparalleled precision in the representations of magnitudes, gradients, and directions of stresses and strains throughout the entire mandible.

The detailed biomechanical events associated with the functional loading of the human mandible are not yet fully fathomed. In general, the methodologies used to record them are extremely invasive. In this regard, computational modeling and simulation offer a promising and alternative approach with the additional capability to predict regional stresses and strains in inaccessible locations. The ability to extract data from computed tomography (CT) or any other appropriate imaging technology to generate the patient's own model is already a common practice. For example, by integrating computerized modeling with medical imaging, it would be possible to determine the correct location, configuration, size and number of implants needed to address the patient's functional and restorative needs. Furthermore, this approach can be used to define the form and mechanical requirements of implants and prostheses employed in the treatment of mandibular and maxillary fractures with fixation and reduction of the fracture obtained with minimal osteosynthesis plate bulk, number and size. This integrated system can be coupled with modern rapid prototyping such as 3D printing and laser sintering to produce superstructures and patient matched dental devices and guides.

In the last section, this book will cover the types of bioceramics and surface modifications currently used in dentistry and oral and maxillofacial surgery as well as their production methods and properties. Bioceramics performed singular and biologically inert roles when utilized as implants prior to the 1970s. The limitations with these synthetic materials as tissue substitutes were highlighted with the growing realization that tissues and cells within the human body performed numerous different vital regulatory and metabolic roles. The demands of bioceramics have changed since then, from maintaining an essentially physical function without eliciting a host response to providing a more positive interaction with the host. This has been accompanied by increasing demands on medical devices that they not only improve the quality of life but also extend its duration. Of even greater importance are the exciting and potential opportunities associated with the use of nanobioceramics as body interactive materials in, helping the body to heal, or promoting the regeneration of tissues, thus restoring physiological functions.

The relationship between biological responses and surface properties of materials is one of the main issues in biomedical materials research. Currently, one of the key drawbacks of synthetic implants is their failure to adapt to the local tissue environment. Improvements in reliability and biocompatibility of implants and prostheses can be achieved through surface modifications. Surface modification of metallic materials using biomaterial thin films and nanocoatings is intended to stimulate bioactivity, biocompatibility and reliability, while at the same time reducing or eliminating corrosion and metal ion release. Important factors in determining the capability and performance of coated implants under physiological environments are their mechanical and adhesion properties. More importantly, computational modeling approaches are vital in the progress of understanding the interfacial behavior between a coating (or thin film) and the substrate material used. The knowledge gained will result in better design and selection of coating and substrate materials.

Andy H. Choi
Faculty of Science
University of Technology Sydney
Australia

ACKNOWLEDGEMENTS

We would like to acknowledge the hard work and efforts of the editorial team at Bentham Science Publishers and in particular Ms. Hira Aftab.

CONFLICT OF INTEREST

The authors declared no conflict of interest regarding the contents of each of the chapters of this book.

DEDICATION

Dedicated to my family, mentor, and to all those who contributed to this endeavor.

CHAPTER 1

Introduction

Abstract: Implants have not always enjoyed a favorable reputation despite the fact that they have been used for many years to support dental prostheses. The function of a dental implant system is to restore dentition by providing a means of transmitting masticatory forces to the mandibular or maxillary bone. The importance of understanding the way in which the stresses and distortion acting in a dental implant and its surrounding bone structure are distributed is of paramount importance in the field of prosthetic replacement where the principal aim is to replace a damaged tooth so that the patient can function effectively. In response to occlusal forces as well as establishing normal dimensions of the peri-implant soft tissues, bone remodeling will take place during the first year of function. Changes in the internal state of stress in bone due to occlusal forces determine whether destructive or constructive bone remodeling will occur. The careful planning of functional occlusal loading can lead to a possible increase in bone-to-implant contact and maintain osseointegration. On the other hand, bone loss and/or component failure can be the result of insufficient load transfer or excessive loading.

Keywords: Bone remodeling, Dental Implants, Minimum success criteria, Osseointegration, Occlusal force, Stress shielding.

Successful replacement of missing teeth is one of the biggest problems faced in the dental profession. Conventional full dentures may not stress bone properly, causing loss of alveolar bone height and inflammation of soft tissues [1 - 8].

Over the past four decades, interest in the use of dental implants has been increasing steadily. This interest has encouraged the development of many new dental systems and different implant designs. Through the application of computer-based models using computer-aided design systems, modern engineering techniques have been utilized to design different types of implants.

Implants have not always enjoyed a favorable reputation despite the fact that they have been used for many years to support dental prostheses. This situation has changed dramatically with the development of endosseous osseointegrated dental implants. They are a useful addition in the management of patients who have missing teeth due to trauma, diseases, or development anomalies, as they are the nearest replacement equivalent to the natural tooth.

Andy H. Choi and Besim Ben-Nissan

At the moment, there are a number of dental implant systems that offer predictable long-term results supported by sound scientific research as well as clinical trials. The clinical success of an implant is largely determined by the manner in which the mechanical stresses are transferred from the implant to the surrounding bone without generating forces of a magnitude that would jeopardize the longevity of implant and prosthesis [9].

The following are some of the basic terminologies used in implant dentistry as described by Palmer in 1999 [5]:

- *Abutment Screw:* A screw used to connect an abutment to the implant.
- *Endosseous Dental Implant*: It is often referred to as a 'fixture' and is the equivalent to 'tooth root'. By definition, it is a device that is inserted into the jawbone (endosseous) to support a dental prosthesis.
- *Implant Abutment*: It is the component that supports the prosthesis and it is connected to the dental implant. Two types of abutments are commonly used in implant dentistry. A healing or temporary abutment can be employed throughout the healing process of the peri-implant soft tissue prior to the selection of a definitive abutment. A transmucosal abutment or TMA is one type of abutment that passes through the mucosa overlying the implant.
- *Osseointegration:* By definition, osseointegration is the direct functional and structural connection between the surface of a load-carrying implant and the ordered, living bone.
- *Single-stage Implant Surgery:* This is the procedure used in non-submerged implant systems. The process involves surgically placing a dental implant and the implant is left exposed to the oral cavity after insertion.
- *Two-stage Implant Surgery:* This is the protocol used in submerged implant systems. It involves the surgical placement of a dental implant which is buried beneath the mucosa. A number of months later, the implant is then exposed through a second surgical procedure.

It is important to establish the success criteria for implant systems, and for implants to be tested in well-controlled clinical trials. The minimum success criteria proposed by Albrektsson *et al.* [10] is listed below:

1. When tested under clinical conditions, an individual and unattached implant is immobile.
2. No peri-implant radiolucency is revealed during radiographic examination.
3. A radiographic vertical bone loss of less than 0.2 mm per annum is recorded after the first year of function.
4. The performance of individual implants is described by the presence of signs and symptoms such as infections, neuropathies, pain, paraesthesia, or the

violation of the inferior dental canal.

5. The implant should satisfy the first four criteria with a minimum success rate of 85% after a five-year observation period and a rate of 80% at the end of a ten-year observation period.

Mobility and its influence on the surrounding bone are the most obvious signs, when an implant system is failing. The function of a dental implant system is to restore dentition by providing a means of transmitting masticatory forces to the mandibular or maxillary bone. The importance of understanding the way in which the stresses and distortion acting in a dental implant and its surrounding bone structure are distributed is of paramount importance in the field of prosthetic replacement where the principal aim is to replace a damaged tooth so that the patient can function effectively.

A number of the criteria described above can be applied to define the overall requirements for an implant system, but they are not as useful in determining the success of individual implants. This is well demonstrated by considering the radiographic criteria.

In response to occlusal forces as well as establishing normal dimensions of the peri-implant soft tissues, bone remodeling will take place during the first year of function. Changes in the internal state of stress in bone due to occlusal forces determine whether destructive or constructive bone remodeling will occur. Disuse atrophy similar to the loss of alveolar crest after the removal of natural teeth may be the result of low stress levels around a dental implant. In contrast, abnormally high stress concentrations in the supporting tissues can cause pressure necrosis, patient discomfort and eventually failure of the implant system [11]. In general, the "ideal" bone is measured against a definite landmark on the implant such as the implant-abutment junction. For that reason, it may differ between implant systems.

Subsequently, it is impossible to measure small changes in bone levels such as 0.2 mm per annum using conventional radiographs, and bone levels are typically believed to be more or less stable. Hence, these specified changes are applicable to the determination of mean or average changes across a large number of implants rather than an individual implant. For instance, a noticeable change of 1 mm or more can occur in very few implants in contrast to the majority, which remained in a steady state, or unchanged.

Furthermore, specifying the requirements needed to constitute failure for an individual implant based on the levels of change over a given period is also problematic. A long period of stability may be the result of a rapid change in bone level. Continuous or progressive bone loss on the other hand is a worrying sign of impending failure. Thus, it can be said that an implant with obvious loss of bone may be assessed as "surviving" instead of "successful".

According to a study by Albrektsson and Sennerby [4], a higher success rate is observed for implant systems such as Branemark® placed in the mandible (approximately 95% success rate) than compared to those placed in the maxilla (between 85 to 90%) after 5 years of implantation.

The initial stability and subsequent function of the implant are greatly influenced by its design [5]. The primary design parameters are:

A. **Implant Shape:** Shapes that are widely used include hollow or solid screws and hollow or solid cylinders. These shapes are designed to provide good stability during the initial stages of implantation as well as maximizing the potential area for osseointegration. Screw-shaped implants also provide sound distribution of load characteristics during function. Even minor alterations in the pitch and size of threads can enhance the initial stability.
B. **Implant Diameter:** A minimum diameter of 3.25 mm is needed to ensure adequate implant strength. Most implants are approximately 4 mm in diameter. The diameter of implants can be as big as 6 mm, which are also available for clinical applications and are considerably stronger. However, they are not so extensively used given the fact that sufficient bone width is not regularly encountered.
C. **Implant Length:** In general, implant lengths are available from 6 mm up to 20 mm. Implant lengths between 8 and 15 mm are frequently used as they correspond quite closely to normal root lengths.
D. **Surface Characteristics:** The extent of surface roughness differs greatly between different implant systems. No definition has been set regarding the optimal surface morphology, and yet, the performance of some may be better under certain conditions. Surfaces that are currently available include grit-blasted, etched, machined, plasma sprayed and micro- and nano-coated. There is the potential to increase the surface contact with bone through an increase in surface roughness; however, this may be at the expense of more surface corrosion and ionic exchange. Moreover, surface roughness can also influence the amount of bacterial contamination on the implant surface, if it becomes exposed within the oral cavity.

At the time of implant placement, its stability is extremely important and it is determined by factors such as implant design in addition to the quality and quantity of the surrounding bone tissue. The alveolar bone resorbs in height and width following the loss of a tooth. Ideally, jawbone quality consisting of a well-formed cortex and densely trabeculated medullary spaces including a good blood supply is the most beneficial for implant treatment. Good initial stability may be offered by bone that is predominately cortical. In this case, extra precaution must be taken during the drilling process to avoid overheating especially for sites that are more than 10 mm in depth as the bone can be easily damaged. In contrast, very poor initial implant stability is offered by bone with a thin or absent cortical layer and sparse trabeculation. Such bone offers very few cells with good osteogenic potential for promoting osseointegration. Furthermore, the quality of bone is compromised by variables such as heavy smoking, irradiation, and infection.

The utilization of a surgical approach that avoids heating the bone can increase the success rate of dental implantation. Damage to bone tissue occurs at a temperature of approximately 47°C after 1 minute. This can be avoided by using copious saline irrigation, slow drilling speed, and successive incrementally larger sharp drills.

Following its installation, it is vital that the implant is not excessively loaded during the early healing phase. Fibrous tissue encapsulation instead of osseointegration will result if movement of the implant within the bone occurs at this stage. In comparison, this is somewhat similar to the healing of a fracture in which stabilization of the bone fragments is of vital importance for promoting union.

At present, determining precisely the optimum period of healing before loading can commence cannot be accurately quantified. Bone quality can be evaluated during the preparation of the implant site by measuring the cutting torque. Resonance frequency analysis has been used to assess the stability of an implant as well as improvements in bone-to-implant contact [5]. This non-invasive tool measures the stiffness across the interface between bone and implant. Under certain circumstances, if the functional forces can be controlled adequately and bone quality is good, it has been demonstrated that immediate loading is consistent with subsequent successful osseointegration [5]. Abutments are connected to the implant following the recommended healing period of approximately three months to allow construction of prosthesis. Thus, this procedure prevents further surgery to uncover the implants.

The careful planning of functional occlusal loading can lead to a possible increase in bone-to-implant contact and maintain osseointegration. On the other hand, bone loss and/or component failure can be the result of insufficient load transfer or excessive loading. Implant overload can arise mainly from two factors: prosthesis design and parafunctional activities. Excessive occlusal forces generated in either or both situations present opportunity for loosening and/or fracture of the screws through bending overload [12]. Bending overload can be defined as a situation in which occlusal forces on an implant-supported prosthesis exert a bending moment resulting from non-axial loading on the implant cross-section at the crestal bone level [13].

CHAPTER 2

Bone Structure

Abstract: From a macroscopic point of view, human bone appears in two forms. The most obvious difference between these two types of bone is their volume fraction of solids or relative densities. The term cortical or compact is used to categorize bone with a volume fraction of solids greater than 70 percent. On the other hand, bone with a volume fraction of solids less than 70 percent is referred to as cancellous or trabecular. Typically, most bones within the human body possess both types: a core of spongy cancellous bone is surrounded by an outer shell composed of a dense compact bone. The constitutive properties of cancellous bone are of vital importance as it is this bone that is in direct contact with the implant or prosthesis.

Keywords: Cortical bone, Cancellous bone, Density, Elastic modulus, Mechanical properties, Nanoindentation, Physical properties, Ultrasonic testing.

Human bone appears in two forms from a macroscopic term of view. The most obvious difference between these two types of bone is their volume fraction of solids or relative densities. The term cortical or compact is used to categorize bone with a volume fraction of solids greater than 70 percent. On the other hand, bone with a volume fraction of solids less than 70 percent is referred to as cancellous or trabecular. Typically, most bones within the human body possess both types: a core of spongy cancellous bone is surrounded by an outer shell composed of a dense compact bone (Fig. **1**).

On a smaller scale, bone is composed of concentric cylinders referred to as a Haversian system as shown in Fig. (**2**). It is a matrix with layers of cells laminated between cylinders. The complete structure can be either loosely packed cancellous bone or densely packed cortical bone.

Both the cortical and cancellous bones are constructed using one-third organic material and two-thirds inorganic material. The inorganic material is principally calcium carbonate and calcium phosphate, while the organic material consists of three different types of cells.

Andy H. Choi and Besim Ben-Nissan

The first type of cells is the osteoblasts, which are commonly thought of as the cells responsible for bone formation. The second type is the osteoclasts and is responsible for the demineralization of bone and in the formation of the matrix. The last type is the fibroblasts, which is responsible for forming collagenous fibers. Both the osteoblasts and osteoclasts are confined within the 'Haversian' and surrounding network. Rodan *et al.* [16] and later Binderman *et al.* [17] suggested that these cells might function as site-specific activators as well as regulators governing the establishment of new bones.

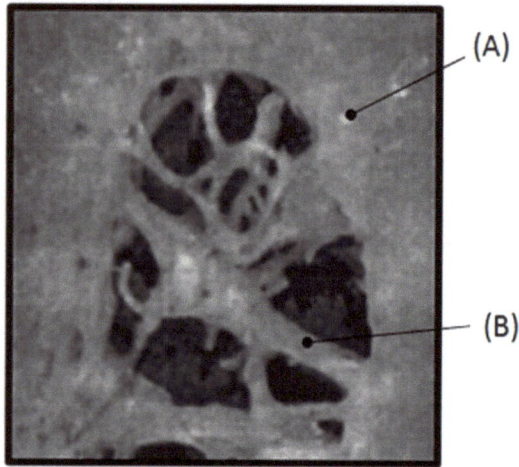

Fig. (1). Cross-section of the mandible showing the cortical bone outline (**A**) and cancellous bone inner layer (**B**). Modified from [14].

Cortical bone can be considered as a multi-component biological composite material consisting of an organic matrix (collagen and protein molecules), water, and mineral phases (crystalline and amorphous hydroxyapatite (HAp)) [18 - 20]. The organic phase mainly contains Type I collagen fibers which possess a number of the characteristics associated with polymeric materials [19]. The mineral phase is mainly comprised of carbonate apatite crystals (CHAP) which precipitate around the collagen fibers [21]. Furthermore, it has been discovered that CHAP exhibited a behavior similar to that of ceramic materials [19]. The water phase, bound and unbound, facilitates the interactions between the organic and mineral phases [22, 23].

From a different perspective, cortical bone can be thought of as a hierarchical solid created from structural elements, which in themselves exhibit a discrete structure [24 - 26]. The structure of cortical bone can be classified as lamellar (lamellae), porous (osteocyte lacunae), fibrous (collagen fibers and osteons) and particulate (CHAP crystallites) based on their relative sizes [26].

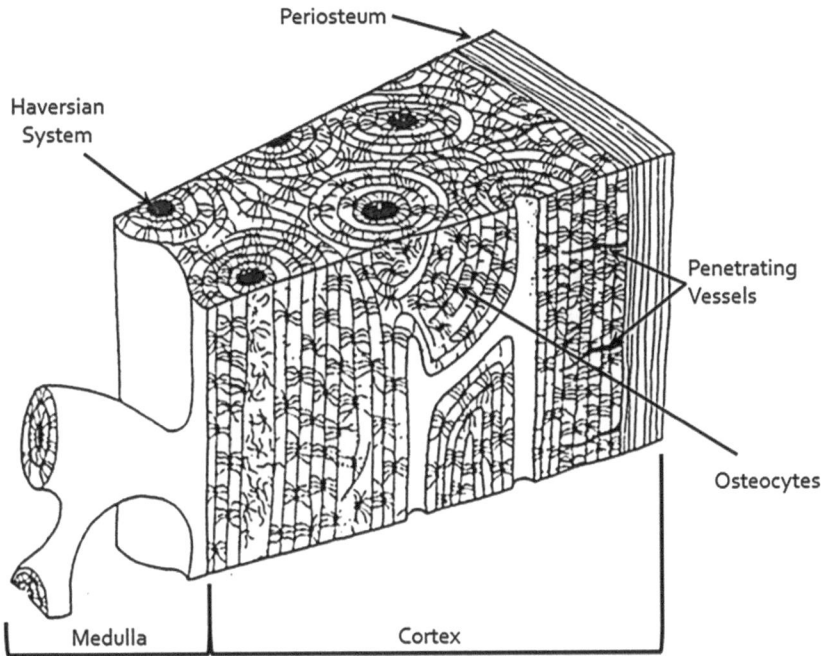

Fig. (2). Bone structure. Modified from [15].

As demonstrated by scanning electron microscopy, the mechanical behavior of cortical bone is dependent on the distribution and sizes of the phases that begins at the elemental (less than 0.005 micron) and microstructural (between 1 to 10 microns) level [27]. At the next level in the hierarchy, which is from 10 to 50 microns, the mechanical behavior of cortical bone can be determined from microhardness testing [28], which measures the physical effects of small-scale changes in the mineral content of the bone [29].

More importantly, nanoindentation has been used to examine the properties of hard tissues such as bone since the 1990s [30 - 36]. This technique allows the measurement of mechanical properties such as hardness and the elastic modulus at the surface of a material. In comparison to other conventional mechanical tests such as tensile testing, the procedure for nanoindentation is much simpler, in particular for small complex-shaped samples such as dentine, cementum and enamel [37]. Importantly, this technique enables the measurement of mechanical properties in a very small selected region within the specimen where the dimensions may be at a micrometer or even nanometer scale, which is essential when measuring local properties of non-homogeneous structures such as dental calcified tissues.

A relationship exists between the mineral fraction and mechanical properties of cortical bone [38 - 41]. Small changes in the mineral fraction will result in a significant change in the material properties.

The constitutive properties of cancellous bone are of vital importance as it is this bone that is in direct contact with the implant or prosthesis. In simple terms, cancellous bone is a cellular material composed of a connected network of plates or rods. A network of plates produces closed cells, while a network of rods creates open cells. Its mechanical behavior is typically a cellular material. With such material, the stress-strain graph has three distinct phases of behavior (Fig. **3**).

In the first phase, the compressive behavior is linear elastic as the cell walls bend or axially compressed. Ultimately, the cells begin to collapse by elastic buckling at high enough loads, which also leads to plastic yielding or brittle fracture of the cell walls. This second phase of collapse proceeds at a roughly constant load until the cell wells meet and touch. The resistance to load increases at this point and this results in the progressively steep final portion of the stress-strain graph as shown in Fig. (**3**).

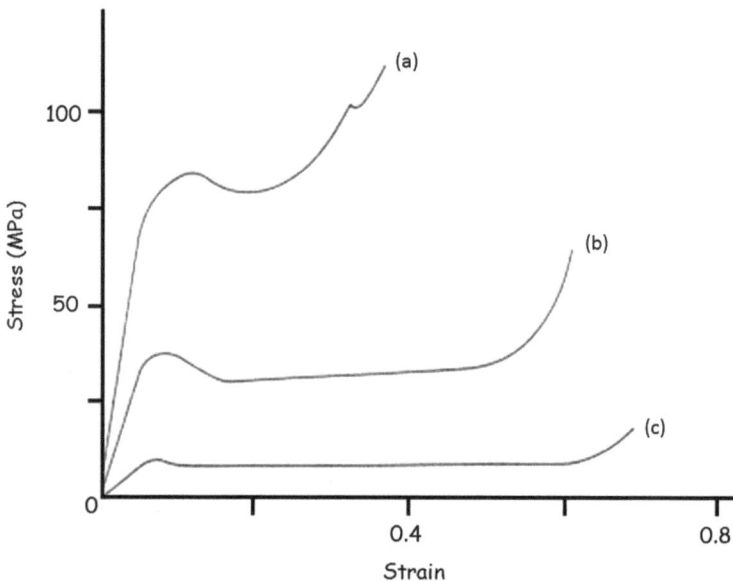

Fig. (3). The compressive behavior of cancellous bone as represented using a stress-strain graph. (**a**) $\rho/\rho_s = 0.5$; (**b**) $\rho/\rho_s = 0.4$; (**c**) $\rho/\rho_s = 0.3$. It can be seen that as the relative density increases, the compressive strength and elastic modulus also increase. Modified from [42].

The direction of the applied load will govern the symmetry of the cancellous bone structure. For instance, if the stress pattern in the cancellous bone is complex, then the structure of the trabeculae network will also become complex and highly asymmetric. On the other hand, in bones such as the vertebrae where the loading is mainly uniaxial, the trabeculae frequently develop a columnar structure with cylindrical symmetry [43, 44].

The orientation of the bone columns is positioned in the vertical direction. This arrangement gives bone a relatively high strength and stiffness in the direction of the applied load and lower strength and stiffness in the transverse directions. As a result, four basic categories of structures are created for cancellous bone:

A. Asymmetric, open cell, rod-like structure;
B. Columnar, open cell, rod-like structure;
C. Asymmetric, closed cell, plate-like structure; and
D. Columnar, closed cell, plate-like structure.

It has been proven, both theoretically and experimentally, that elastic modulus of cancellous bone is strongly dependent on the structural density, or sometimes referred to as the apparent density, of bone [45 - 50].

Within a number of areas in the human skeleton, cancellous bone retains a structure with unique textural anisotropy. Consequently, the properties of cancellous bone cannot be predicted accurately using a single scalar measurement such as structural or apparent density. The elastic constants of cancellous bone in such instances are determined by its structural density as well as its textural anisotropy.

There have been a number of experimental studies in recent years on determining the elastic properties of bone. Most of these efforts have focused on long bones, and in particular, the femur. One of the principal findings of these investigations is that the elastic properties of bone differ with both the orientation and position of the specimen. In other words, bone is both anisotropic and heterogeneous in its elastic properties.

Given the fact that bone is an anisotropic and heterogeneous material, the anatomical location of the specimen will have an influence on the experimental results. The standard parameters of the type of experiment carried out, such as the duration of load and deformation rate in mechanical tests or vibrational frequency in ultrasonic tests, will also affect the results obtained.

The mechanical characteristics of bone vary with the types of bone, biological variables such as age, gender and race, its possible state of pathological degradation, levels of activity of the living bone, along with the preservation conditions of the specimen up until the time of experimentation, all of which contribute to the irregular distribution of its mechanical properties [51].

2.1. PHYSICAL AND MECHANICAL PROPERTIES

Forces are applied to the mandible through the teeth, the muscles of mastication, and through reaction forces at the temporomandibular joints. In order to fully comprehend the reaction of the mandible to the applied force, it is essential to gain an in-depth understanding of how the internal forces are distributed throughout the entire mandible and how the mandible deforms as a consequence of those internal forces.

The internal force intensity at a particular point is described by the six independent components of stress, and the deformation in the neighborhood of a point is characterized by the six independent components of strain. The six components are:

1. x_{11};
2. x_{22};
3. x_{33};
4. x_{23};
5. x_{13}; and
6. x_{12}.

where x represents a component of stress or strain, and the numbers 1, 2, and 3 represents the radial, circumferential, and axial directions, respectively (Fig. **4**).

The components of stress are related to the components of strain through a constitutive relation. The constitutive relation appears to be adequate for bone when it is considered as an inhomogeneous, anisotropic, linearly elastic material [52].

Data on the material properties of mandibular cortical and cancellous bone have been determined on small specimens obtained from human tibiae and from the mandibles of cadavers and humans by means of ultrasonic wave techniques and material testing techniques [30 - 36, 53 - 69]. With respect to the material properties of the cancellous bone of the mandible, limited data are available.

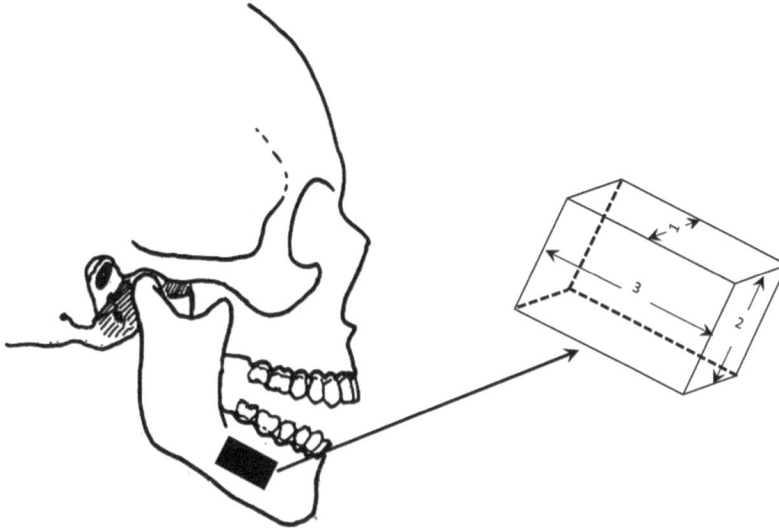

Fig. (4). Definition of directions. 1: direction is radial or normal to the surface of the bone; 2: direction is tangential or supero-inferior along the bone surface; 3: longitudinal or axial along the bone surface.

The utilization of ultrasonic waves is a well-known technique for determining the elastic properties of bone. The elastic properties can be deduced from velocity measurements of shear and longitudinal waves propagating in particular directions in the bone specimens if the density and the elastic anisotropy of bone are specified.

It should be mentioned that the properties of mandibular cortical bone are generally determined in three orthogonal directions relative to the surface of each sample: longitudinal, radial and tangential (Fig. **4**). A limitation of the loading experiments is that loading could not be performed in the radial direction because of the overall cortical thickness in this direction [65, 66]. As a result, the elastic constants and yield stresses for the radial direction are estimated from those obtained from the tangential direction.

The values of elastic constants reported in a number of studies are summarized in Table **1**. Based on the results of these studies, it can be clearly seen that the cortical bone of the mandible behaves in an anisotropic manner. This implies that it is stiffer in the longitudinal than in the tangential and radial directions. The average elastic moduli in the longitudinal direction are approximately 40% - 70% higher than those of the radial and tangential directions. Moreover, the elastic moduli in the radial and tangential directions have about the same values. Consequently, the cortical bone of the mandible can be considered as transversely isotropic, with a higher elastic modulus in the longitudinal direction and a lower elastic modulus in all transverse directions. The strength of the mandible is also higher in longitudinal than in transverse directions.

Table 1. Elastic modulus (E), shear modulus (G), and Poisson's ratio (v) of the human mandible. The 1-direction is radial, the 2-direction is circumferential and the 3-direction is longitudinal. The values of E and G are displayed in GPa [54, 57, 65 - 66, 69].

	Arendts and Sigolotto	Ashman and Van Buskirk	Carter	Dechow *et al.*
E_1	6.9	10.8	13.0	11.3
E_2	8.2	13.3	13.0	13.8
E_3	17.3	19.4	19.0	19.4
G_{12}		3.81	5.3	4.5
G_{13}		4.12	5.9	5.2
G_{23}		4.63	5.9	6.2
v_{12}	0.270	0.309	0.22	0.274
v_{13}	0.125	0.249	0.29	0.237
v_{21}	0.150	0.381	0.22	0.317
v_{23}	0.325	0.224	0.29	0.273
v_{31}	0.310	0.445	0.42	0.405
v_{32}	0.315	0.328	0.42	0.376

Based on the results of their findings, Arendts and Sigolotto [65, 66] have suggested that the mandible is stronger and stiffer in the longitudinal direction could be the result of the orientation of osteons, apatite crystals, and collagen fibers. Using a material testing approach, the mean yield compressive stresses of 100, 110, and 200 MPa and strain values at the yield points of 2.25%, 2.05%, and 1.55% in the radial, tangential, and longitudinal directions, respectively were obtained from specimens taken at various regions of three mandibles. Similar observations were also made in an earlier study by Bacon *et al.* [70], where they reported the relationship between the orientations of apatite crystals and muscle attachments in the mandible.

In 1987, Ashman and Van Buskirk described the human mandibular bone as elastically homogeneous but anisotropic [54]. Parallelepiped specimens were taken from ten different locations in the human mandible, and their elastic properties were determined using a continuous-wave ultrasonic technique. Data on the elastic properties revealed that the mandible behaves in a manner similar to that of a slightly less stiff long bone that is bent into the shape of a horseshoe. Later, the elastic and shear modulus as well as Poisson's ratio of 17 mandibles were also determined in a study by Dechow *et al.* using ultrasonic wave techniques [57]. An average density of 1.768 g/cc was recorded from the mandible samples. The densities of each sample were determined using the Archimedes Principle of buoyancy method.

As mentioned earlier, nanoindentation is another approach that can be used to evaluate the elastic properties of human bone at a microstructural level. However, as mentioned in a study by Turner *et al.* [31], nanoindentation may produce inaccurate results due to the fact that the technique calculates the elastic modulus of a material with the assumption that it behaves in an elastically isotropic manner. To demonstrate that nanoindentation can potentially be used to measure the elastic properties of anisotropic bone, they compared the elastic moduli of bone tissue from a common human donor measured using acoustic microscopy to those measured using nanoindentation. Their findings showed the elastic modulus of cortical bone in the longitudinal direction was about 40% greater than that in the transverse direction. More importantly, the nanoindentation technique estimated elastic moduli that were 4% - 14% higher than those measured using acoustic microscopy (Table **2**). However, the average anisotropy ratio (the elastic modulus in the longitudinal or axial direction divided by the elastic modulus in the transverse direction) for cortical bone determined by the acoustic microscope (1.39) was similar to that determined by nanoindentation (1.41)

Table 2. Elastic Modulus of cortical bone (in GPa) determined using nanoindentation and acoustic measurement techniques [31]. (Note: data is reported as mean ± standard deviation).

Specimen	E (Nanoindentation)	E (Acoustic)
Cortical Bone (*Longitudinal*)	23.45 ± 0.21	20.55 ± 0.21
Cortical Bone (*Transverse*)	16.58 ± 0.32	14.91 ± 0.52

The abovementioned work discusses the elastic properties of cortical bone. A number of studies were also carried out to determine the properties of cancellous bone at specific sites throughout the human mandible and of other human bones such as the tibiae. In 1990, the elastic properties of cancellous bone were measured using ultrasonic technique [71]. The structural density of 75 specimens from three human proximal tibiae ranged from 0.109 to 0.768 g/cc (Table **3**). The apparent density as well as elastic properties of the cancellous structures was also quantified in a study by Rho using ultrasonic techniques [58]. Eight tibiae were obtained from frozen human cadavers taken from the right side of eight individuals. One hundred and forty four cancellous bone specimens were obtained from the proximal tibiae. The apparent density of the cancellous structure ranged from 50 to 1000 kg/m^3, which was determined by weighing the cancellous structure after removing the bone marrow divided by the volume of the overall physical dimensions, including pores. The porosity of cancellous bone induces variations of apparent densities over several orders of magnitudes.

Table 3. Elastic modulus (E), shear modulus (G), and Poisson's ratio (v) of human tibial cancellous bone. The 1-direction is radial, the 2-direction is circumferential and the 3-direction is longitudinal. The values of E and G are displayed in MPa [58, 71]. (Note: standard deviation in parentheses).

	Turner *et al.*	Rho
E_1	316.7	202 (154)
E_2	385.5	232 (180)
E_3	959.3	769 (534)
G_{12}	88.7	
G_{13}	125.6	
G_{23}	165.7	
v_{12}		
v_{13}		
v_{21}		
v_{23}	0.3	
v_{31}	0.3	
v_{32}	0.3	

Using an edentulous human mandible, the values of elastic modulus of cancellous bone were determined in three orthogonal directions by means of compression testing of cubes cut with the faces aligned with the anatomic axes [67]. Samples were kept moist with buffered saline and tested in each of the three directions of the cube (Table **4**). Using the same test samples, investigations were also carried out to determine bone mass and volume fraction following mechanical testing. Samples were defatted in absolute alcohol for 3 days, blown free of remaining marrow with an air jet, and dried in air for 24 hours. Bone area fraction was measured directly under light microscopy from the two faces perpendicular to the mesio-distal axis using the line-intercept method. Bone volume fraction averaged 0.33 and apparent density averaged 0.55 g/cc. Elastic modulus was greatest in the mesio-distal direction (mean 907 MPa), followed by the bucco-lingual (mean 511 MPa) and infero-superior direction (mean 114 MPa). This suggests a model of transverse isotropy for cancellous bone in the jaw, where the symmetry axis is along the infero-superior (weakest) direction.

Table 4. Physical and mechanical properties of cancellous bone based on anatomical sites [67].

Anatomic Sites	Apparent Density (g/cc)	Elastic Modulus, E (MPa)		
		Infero-Superior	Bucco-Lingual	Mesio-Distal
Left central incisor	0.30	56	126	52
Left lateral incisor	0.40	105	160	312
Right central incisor	0.98	123	1113	2283
Right canine	0.23	48	71	140
Right first premolar (interior)	0.75	262	1464	1768
Right second premolar (superior)	0.78	158	553	805
Right second premolar	0.39	47	91	988

2.2. REGIONAL VARIATIONS

Despite the fact that the yield strength and elastic moduli measured in the studies by Arendts and Sigolotto showed regional variation [65, 66], that is, up to a factor of 1.5 between minimum and maximum values, their data do not point to systematic differences between particular locations of the mandible (for example, corpus *vs.* ramus, lower margin *vs.* upper margin). In contrast, a study by Dechow *et al.* [56] discovered that the stiffest region of the mandibular corpus is located at the lower border inferior to the canine. According to these authors, this region is capable of withstanding high levels of torsion and it is in this region where torsional stresses are suspected to change during functional movements. Table **5** summarizes the values of elastic constants of human cortical bone reported in different regions of the human body.

In addition, findings from two other studies [59, 72] showed the following:

A. The cortical bone is stiffer at the lower border of the corpus than at the alveolus;
B. The longitudinal elastic modulus is higher in the symphysis region than in the molar region; and
C. The lingual cortex is stiffer than the buccal cortex in the symphysis and premolar regions.

Compared to the molar region in the body of the mandible, a higher longitudinal elastic modulus at the symphysis may compensate for the suggested larger torsional loadings experienced in that area. Supporting this notion are the numbers on the apparent and mineralization densities revealing that the regions with the highest density are located at the symphysis [73, 74].

Table 5. Elastic modulus (E), shear modulus (G), and Poisson's ratio (v) of human cortical bone measured at different locations. The 1-direction is radial, the 2-direction is circumferential, and the 3-direction is axial. The values of E and G are displayed in GPa [57, 58 - 60]. (Note: standard deviation in parentheses).

	Tibiae	Supraorbital Bone	Parietal Bone
E_1	11.7 (1.3)	10.9 (3.1)	11.8 (2.1)
E_2	12.2 (1.4)	15.2 (4.5)	13.7 (3.1)
E_3	20.7 (1.9)	15.2 (3.5)	19.6 (3.8)
G_{12}	4.1 (0.5)	3.9 (1.3)	4.0 (0.8)
G_{13}	5.2 (0.6)	3.9 (1.1)	4.5 (0.9)
G_{23}	5.7 (0.5)	5.2 (1.1)	6.4 (1.0)
v_{12}	0.420 (0.074)	0.278 (0.087)	0.435 (0.150)
v_{13}	0.237 (0.041)	0.264 (0.113)	0.205 (0.085)
v_{21}	0.231 (0.035)	0.376 (0.093)	0.475 (0.095)
v_{23}	0.435 (0.057)	0.229 (0.048)	0.190 (0.080)
v_{31}	0.417 (0.048)	0.357 (0.139)	0.320 (0.120)
v_{32}	0.390 (0.021)	0.244 (0.088)	0.265 (0.095)

The elastic properties obtained from the human supraorbital region [57], parietal bone [60], human femur [54], and the human tibiae [58] using the ultrasonic technique were compared with the properties of the human mandible as shown in Table **1**. Comparisons of material properties of mandibular bone tissue with those of the supraorbital region [57] indicate that bone from the mandible along the longitudinal axis is stiffer than bone from the supraorbital region. Comparison of material properties of mandibular bone tissue with those of the human tibiae [58] and the parietal bone [60] shows roughly similar values.

CHAPTER 3

Functional Anatomy of the Skull

Abstract: The masticatory system is the functional unit of the body primarily responsible for chewing, speaking and swallowing. The system is made up of bones, joints, ligaments, teeth and muscles. The system of mastication is a highly refined and complex unit. Gaining an in-depth knowledge into its biomechanics and functional anatomy is necessary to the study of occlusion. The mandible is a horseshoe-shaped bone supporting the lower teeth and makes up the lower portion of the facial skeleton. It is suspended below the maxilla by ligaments, other soft tissues, and muscles, which provide the mobility required to function with the maxilla. The energy that moves the mandible and allows function of the masticatory system is provided by muscles. There are four pairs of muscles (left and right side of the mandible) that make up a group known as the muscles of mastication.

Keywords: Cranium, Dentition, Lateral pterygoid, Ligaments, Maxilla, Mandible, Muscles of mastication, Masseter, Mandibular movement, Medial pterygoid, Tooth, Temporomandibular joint, TMJ, Temporalis.

The masticatory system is the functional unit within the human body, whose primary responsibility is chewing, swallowing and speaking. The system is composed of teeth, ligaments, bones, muscles and joints. Furthermore, there is a complex neurologic controlling system that coordinates as well as regulates all these structural constituents [75].

3.1. TOOTH AND DENTITION

Each human tooth can be separated into two basic sections. The root is buried and surrounded by the alveolar bone. The attachment between the roots of teeth to the alveolar bone is made using many fibers of connective tissue which extends from the cementum surface of the root to the alveolar bone. Most of these fibers span diagonally from the cementum in a cervical direction of the bone. The other section of the human tooth is the crown, which is visible above the gingival tissue [75].

As a group, these connective tissue fibers are commonly known as periodontal ligaments. In addition to firmly attaching the tooth to its bony socket, the perio-

Andy H. Choi and Besim Ben-Nissan

dontal ligament also plays a vital role in the dissipation of forces applied to the bone through contacts with the teeth during functional movements such as clenching.

The human dentition consists of 32 permanent teeth which are equally distributed in the alveolar bone of the mandibular and maxillary arches. The maxillary arch is somewhat larger than the mandibular arch. During occlusion, this results in the overlapping of the teeth in the maxilla and mandible both horizontally and vertically.

A greater arch width is the consequence of the maxillary frontal teeth being much wider than the mandibular teeth. Furthermore, anterior tooth in the maxilla have larger facial angulation than compared to those in the mandible, creating a vertical and horizontal overlapping [75].

3.2. CRANIUM

The human cranium or skull is the bony structure which forms the head in the human skeleton and is composed of many bones closely fitted together. Except for the mandible and the ossicles of the middle ear, the bones of the adult skull are joined by rigid structures of synchondroses. The skull is composed of 22 separate bone pieces. A united single and immobile entity are created using 21 of 22 bone segments. The mandible or the lower jaw is the only movable bone within the skull. It is also the last segment of the cranium.

The cranium plays two vital roles in the skeletal structure: firstly, the brain is protected, and secondly, the face is supported by the skull. The skull can be divided into two parts: neurocranium and the facial skeleton.

The neurocranium or commonly referred to as the braincase or cranial-vault contains the inner and middle ear structures. It also encloses and protects the brain. It is constructed using eight bones including the ethmoid bone, frontal bone, the occipital bone, the sphenoid, two parietal bones, and two temporal bones.

The facial bones support the teeth of the upper and lower jaws, surround the eyeball, create the nasal cavity, and provide the basis for the facial constructions. Fourteen bones are involved in the formation of the facial skeleton. These include two maxilla, two palatine bones, two zygomatic bones, two nasal conchae, two lacrimal bones, two nasal bones, the vomer and the mandible.

The maxilla, or often referred to as the upper jaw, is formed by the fusion of two irregularly shaped maxillary bone at the palatal suture, which is located at the mid-line of the roof of the mouth. Each half of the fused bones contains four processes: zygomatic, frontal, palatine and alveolar processes of the maxilla. These bones form the greater portion of the upper facial skeleton (Fig. **5**).

The floor of the nasal cavity in addition to the floor of each orbit is formed as the border of the maxilla extends superiorly. Conversely, the alveolar ridge and the palate is created as the maxillary bone is extended inferiorly, which support 16 maxillary teeth. These teeth are aligned in the alveolar process of the maxilla, which is fixed to the lower anterior portion of the skull. These teeth are aligned in the alveolar process of the maxilla and it is fixed to the lower anterior portion of the skull.

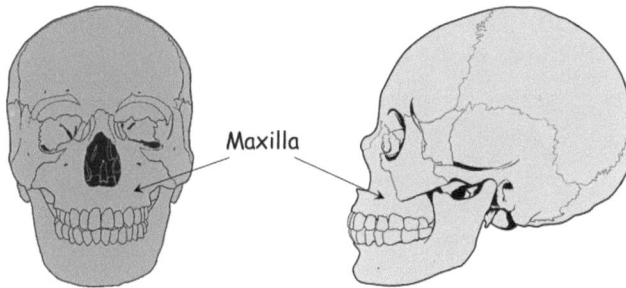

Fig. (5). Anterior and lateral aspect of the skull and the location of the maxilla. Modified from [76].

On the inferior skull, the palatine process from each maxillary bone is fused together to create the anterior portion of the hard palate. The hard palate, created from palatine bone, is a bony plate which separates the nasal cavity from the oral cavity by forming the floor of the nasal cavity and the roof of the mouth. The palatine bone is one of a pair of irregularly shaped bones that have made a small contribution to the formation of the medial wall of each orbit and the lateral wall of the nasal cavity. The horizontal plate is the largest region of each of the palatine bone.

In the maxilla, the zygomatic process grows in a lateral direction until it reaches the zygomatic bone. Also known as the cheekbone, the zygomatic bone is paired to construct most of the lateral wall of the orbit and the lateral-inferior boundaries of the anterior orbital opening. Projecting posteriorly, the short temporal process of the zygomatic bone forms the anterior portion of the zygomatic arch.

The temporal bone is found directly underneath the temple and forms the lower lateral side of the cranium. The temporal bone is divided into a number of sections. The squama temporalis is located in the upper portion of the temporal bone. It has a flat and scale-like appearance. More importantly, it is also where the temporalis muscles are attached (Fig. **6**). The zygomatic process of the temporal bone is located below the squama temporalis and protruding anteriorly. This also creates the posterior section of the zygomatic arch.

The mastoid portion is rougher and heavier and is located posterior to the temporal bone. The mastoid process, projected from the inferior section of the mastoid portion, is a large bulge that can be felt easily behind the earlobe on the side of the head. It also serves as a site for muscle attachment (Fig. **7**).

With each temporal bone, the petrous portion forms a protruding and diagonally oriented petrous ridge in the floor of the cranial cavity. It is, by far the hardest piece of the temporal and it fuses together the inner pieces of squama and mastoid temporalis segments of the temporal bone. Another function of the petrous ridge is the housing of structures of the inner and middle ears.

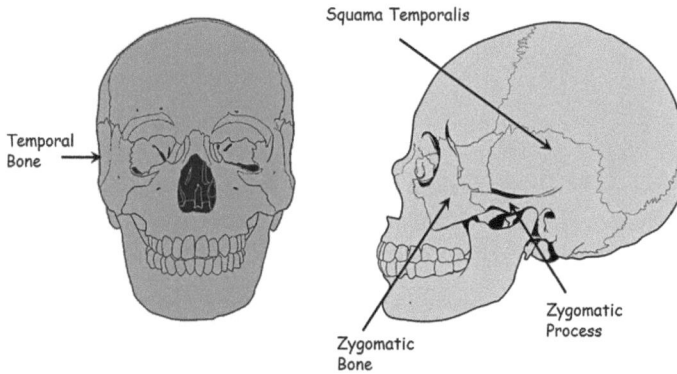

Fig. (6). Temporal bone and the locations of squama temporalis, the zygomatic bone, and zygomatic process. Modified from [76].

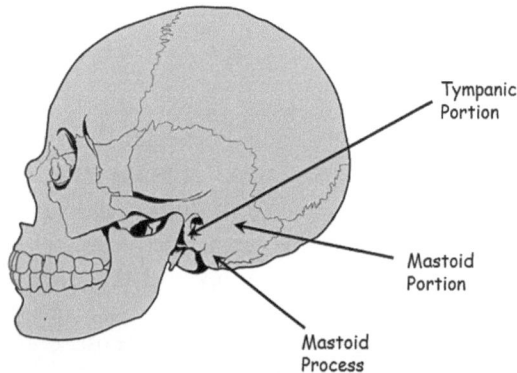

Fig. (7). The locations of the mastoid portion, mastoid process, and the tympanic portion. Modified from [76].

3.3. MANDIBLE

The mandible is a horseshoe-shaped bone supporting the lower teeth and makes up the lower portion of the facial skeleton. It is suspended below the maxilla by ligaments, other soft tissues, and muscles, which provide the mobility required to function with the maxilla (Fig. **8**).

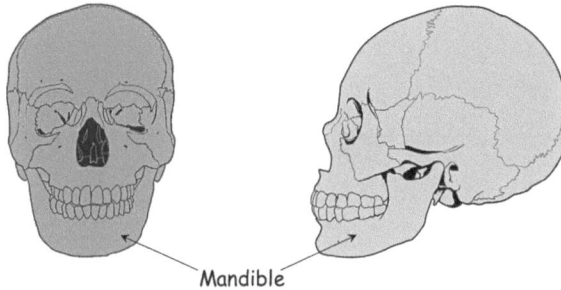

Fig. (8). The mandible. Modified from [76].

The inferior margin of the body meets the posterior margin of the ramus at the angle of the mandible. This area is irregular, being the site of insertion of the masseter muscle and stylomandibular ligament. The junction of the alveolus and ramus is demarcated by a ridge of bone, the external oblique line, which continues downwards and forwards across the body of the mandible, terminating below the mental foramen (Fig. **9**).

The coronoid and the condyle processes form the two processes of the superior border of the ramus.

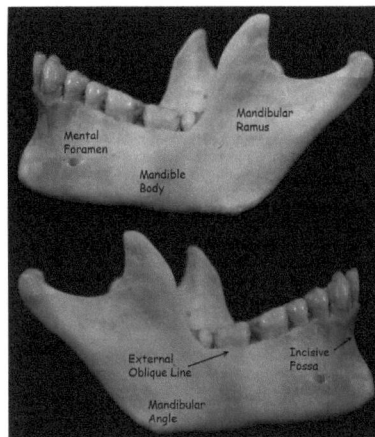

Fig. (9). Features of the mandible. Modified from [77].

The coronoid process provides attachment for the temporalis muscle. The condylar process has a neck supporting an articular surface, which fits into the glenoid fossa of the temporal bone to form a movable synovial joint, the temporomandibular joint (Fig. **10**).

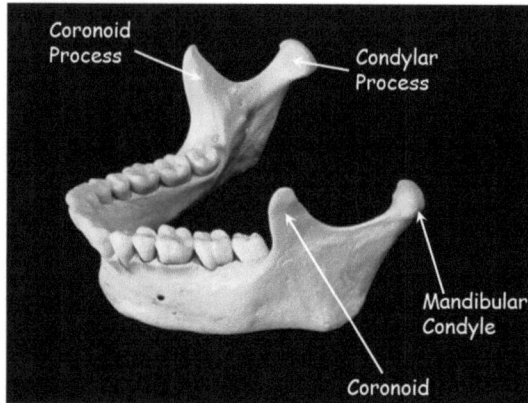

Fig. (10). The ascending ramus extends upward to form the coronoid process and the condyle [75].

3.4. TEMPOROMANDIBULAR JOINT (TMJ)

The area where craniomandibular articulation occurs is called the temporomandibular joint (TMJ). The temporomandibular joint is by far the most complex joint in the body. It provides for hinging movement in one plane. However, at the same time it also provides for gliding movements.

The temporomandibular joint is formed by the mandibular condyle fitting into the mandibular fossa of the temporal bone. Separating these two bones from direct articulation is the articular disc. The articular disc is composed of dense fibrous connective tissue devoid of any blood vessels or nerve fibers. Based on its thickness, the articular disc can be subdivided in the sagittal plane into three regions (Fig. **11**). The intermediate zone is the central area of the disc and it is also the thinnest. The disc becomes considerably thicker both posteriorly and anteriorly to the intermediate zone. The articular surface of the condyle is located on the intermediate zone of the disc in the normal joint, surrounded by the thicker anterior and posterior regions.

During mandibular movement, the disc is somewhat flexible and can adapt to the functional demands of the articular surfaces. The disc maintains its morphology unless destructive forces or structural changes occur in the joint. If these changes occur, the morphology of the disc can be irreversibly altered.

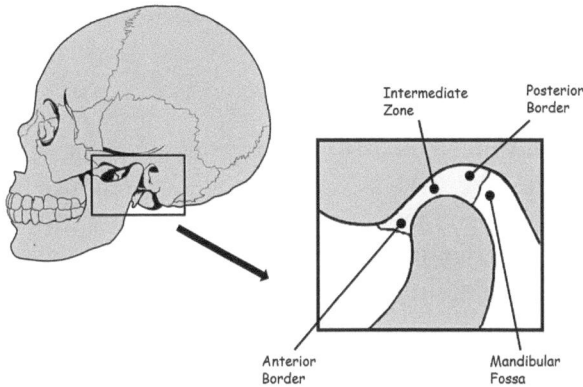

Fig. (11). The temporomandibular joint, mandibular fossa, and the articulating joint [75].

The articular disc is attached posteriorly to an area of loose connective tissue which is innervated and highly vascularized. This is referred to as the retrodiscal tissue. The superior retrodiscal lamina primarily consists of elastic fibers. On the other hand, the inferior retrodiscal lamina is mainly made up of collagenous fibers (Fig. **12**).

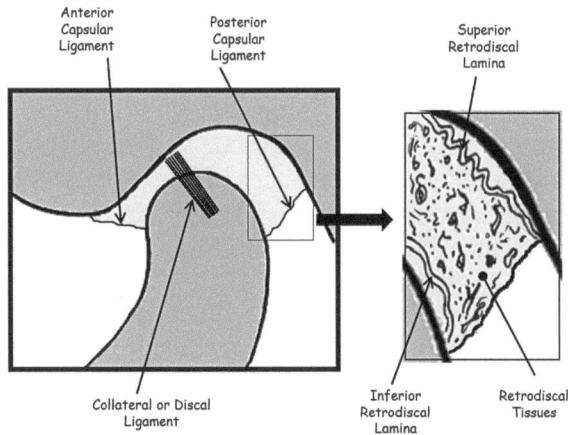

Fig. (12). Lateral aspect of the temporomandibular joint [75].

A synovial lining is formed by the internal surfaces of the cavities that are surrounded by specialized endothelial cells. Synovial fluid is produced by this lining together with a specialized synovial fringe situated at the anterior border of the retrodiscal tissues.

This synovial fluid performs two functions. The synovial fluid serves as a medium for providing metabolic requirements to these tissues as the articular surfaces of the joint are nonvascular. The synovial fluid also acts as a lubricant between articular surfaces during function.

There are two different mechanisms in which the articular surfaces are lubricated by the synovial fluid. The first is termed boundary lubrication and this occurs when synovial fluid is forced from one area of the cavity into another during joint movement. A second lubricating mechanism is referred to as weeping lubrication and this implies to the capability of the reticular surfaces to absorb a small amount of synovial fluid.

Supporting the temporomandibular joint are three functional ligaments and two accessory ligaments (Fig. **12**). The ligaments are comprised of collagenous connective tissues and they do not stretch. More importantly, the ligaments do not actively participate in joint function but serve as passive restraining mechanisms instead to limit and restrict movement of the joint.

The three functional ligaments are:

1. Capsular ligaments;
2. Collateral ligaments; and
3. Temporomandibular ligaments.

The anterior and posterior capsular ligaments surround and encase the entire temporomandibular joint, thus entrapping the synovial fluid. The ligaments also serve as a resistance to any inferior, lateral, and medial forces which tend to dislocate and separate the articular surfaces. The fibers of the capsular ligaments (both anterior and superior) are attached superiorly to the temporal bone along the borders of the articular surfaces of mandibular fossa and articular eminence [75].

The function of the collateral or discal ligaments is to restrict movement of the articular disc away from the condyle. Hence, they are responsible for the hinging movement of the temporomandibular joint. The collateral ligaments do not stretch and are comprised of collagenous connective tissue fibers. The ligaments join the pole of the condyle to the lateral and medial borders of the articular disc (Fig. **12**).

The temporomandibular ligament consists of two components. The inner horizontal component of the ligament restricts posterior movement of the articular disc and the condyle, while the oblique component prevents excessive dropping of the condyle. Consequently, an important function of the oblique component of the temporomandibular ligament is to regulate the extent of mouth opening. Furthermore, the oblique component also has an effect during normal opening of the jaw. During opening, the mandible can be easily rotated until the teeth are between 20 to 25 mm apart. A distinct change in the opening movement will take place if the mandible opens wider. This signifies the change from the condyle rotating about a fixed point to moving forward and down the articular eminence [75].

The two accessory ligaments are:

1. Sphenomandibular ligament; and
2. Stylomandibular ligament.

The sphenomandibular ligament does not have any significance in terms of restricting mandibular movement. The ligament originates from the spine of the sphenoid bone and extends in a downward and lateral direction to the lingual, which is a small bony prominence located on the medial surface of the mandibular ramus. The role of the stylomandibular ligament is to limit the amount of protrusive mandibular movement. Its origin lies in the styloid process and it terminates at the angle and posterior border of the mandibular ramus [75].

3.5. MUSCLES OF MASTICATION

The energy that moves the mandible and allows function of the masticatory system is provided by muscles. There are four pairs of muscles (left and right side of the mandible) that make up a group known as the muscles of mastication. The muscles of mastication include:

1. Masseter;
2. Temporalis;
3. Medial Pterygoid;
4. Lateral Pterygoid; and
5. Digastric.

The muscles involved in jaw movements such as opening, closing, and protruding include the muscles of mastication and also other muscles, namely suprahyoid and infrahyoid groups.

3.5.1. Masseter

The masseter is made up of two portions or heads: the superficial and deep portion. As fibers of the masseter contract, the mandible is elevated and the teeth are brought into contact (Fig. **13**).

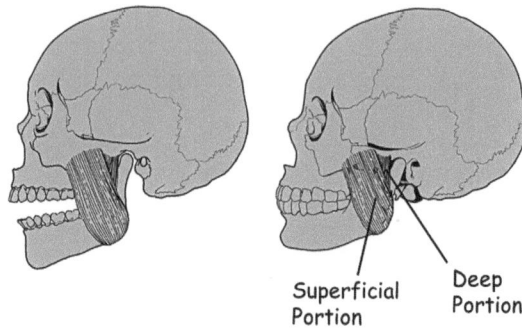

Fig. (13). The masseter muscle. As the muscle contracts, the mandible is elevated [75].

3.5.2. Temporalis

The temporalis is a large fan-shaped muscle. It can be divided into three distinct areas according to fiber direction and ultimate function (Fig. **14**). When the entire temporalis contracts, it elevates the mandible, and the teeth are brought into contact. Because the angulation of its muscle fibers varies, the temporalis is capable of coordinating closing movements. It is thus a significant positioning muscle of the mandible.

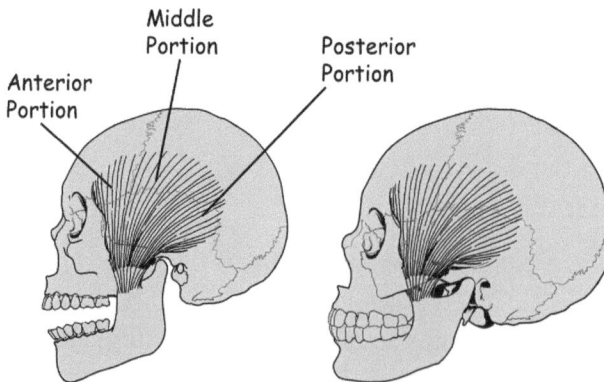

Fig. (14). The temporalis muscle. As the muscle contracts, the mandible is elevated. The exact movement is determined by the location of the fibers being activated [75].

3.5.3. Medial (Internal) Pterygoid

The medial pterygoid muscle, which is situated on the medial side of the mandibular ramus, is a counterpart of the masseter muscle (Fig. **15**), both anatomically and functionally. When its fibers contract, the mandible is elevated and the teeth are brought into contact. This muscle is also active in protruding the mandible.

3.5.4. Lateral (External) Pterygoid

The lateral pterygoid has been described as having two distinct portions: an inferior and a superior. The mandible protrudes when the inferior lateral pterygoid contracts. The mandible is lowered when this muscle functions with the mandibular depressors. The superior lateral pterygoid is especially active during chewing and when the teeth are held together (Fig. **16**).

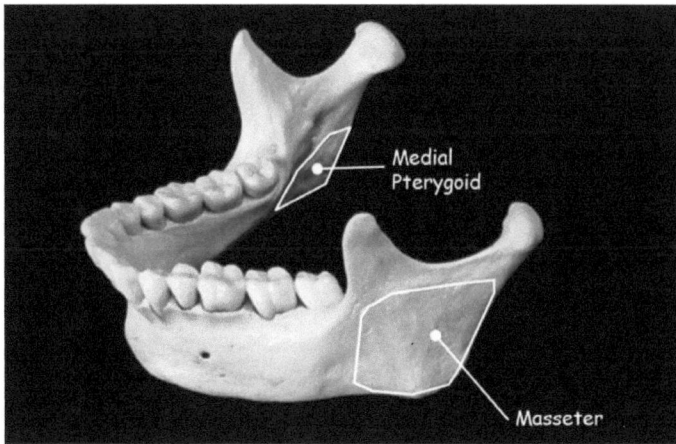

Fig. (15). The locations of muscle insertions for the medial pterygoid and masseter.

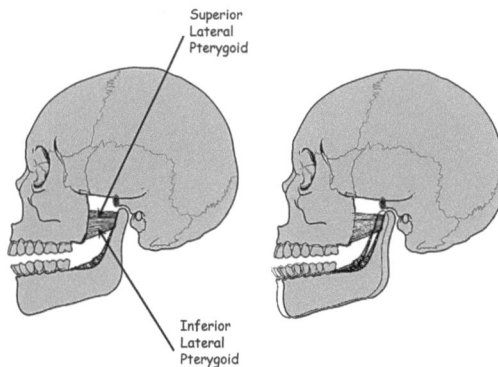

Fig. (16). Superior and inferior lateral pterygoid muscles. The inferior lateral pterygoid muscle is responsible for the protrusion of the mandible [75].

3.5.5. Other Muscles (The Digastric Muscle)

In general, the digastric muscle is not considered as muscles of mastication. However, they do have an important effect on the function of the mandible. The digastric muscle lies beneath the body of the mandible.

The digastric muscle is composed of two muscular bellies (anterior and posterior) connected by an intermediate rounded tendon. The anterior belly ascends from the digastric fossa of mandible, a depression on the inner side of the lower border of the mandible, close to the symphysis, and passes downward and backward. Longer than the anterior belly, the posterior belly ascends from the mastoid notch located on the inferior surface of the skull and medial to the mastoid process of the temporal bone.

The digastric muscle belongs to the suprahyoid muscles group. The digastric is one of the many muscles which depress the mandible and raise the hyoid bone. When the right and left digastric muscles contract, the mandible is depressed and pulled backward and the teeth are brought out of contact.

CHAPTER 4

Introduction

Abstract: The masticatory system is the functional unit of the body primarily responsible for chewing, speaking and swallowing. The system is made up of bones, joints, ligaments, teeth and muscles. The system of mastication is a highly refined and complex unit. Gaining an in-depth knowledge into its biomechanics and functional anatomy is necessary to the study of occlusion. The mandible is a horseshoe-shaped bone supporting the lower teeth and makes up the lower portion of the facial skeleton. It is suspended below the maxilla by ligaments, other soft tissues, and muscles, which provide the mobility required to function with the maxilla. The energy that moves the mandible and allows function of the masticatory system is provided by muscles. There are four pairs of muscles (left and right side of the mandible) that make up a group known as the muscles of mastication.

Keywords: Articular disc, Biomechanics, Chewing stroke, Condyle, Forces of mastication, Mastication, Temporomandibular joint, TMJ, Tooth contact.

The masticatory system is a complex and highly refined unit. A sound understanding of its functional anatomy and biomechanics is essential to the study of occlusion.

4.1. BIOMECHANICS OF THE TEMPOROMANDIBULAR JOINT

The temporomandibular joint is a compound joint. Its structure and function can be divided into two distinct systems:

1. The first system is related to the tissues encasing the inferior synovial cavity. Given the fact that the collateral or discal ligaments tightly attach the articular disc to the condyle, the only physiological movement that can take place between these surfaces is rotation of the disc on the articular surface of the condyle. For this reason, the articular disc-condyle arrangement is the joint structure accountable for the rotational movement within the temporomandibular joint.
2. The second system is related to the articular disc-condyle arrangement as described above, functioning against the surface of the mandibular fossa. Free

sliding movement can occur between these surfaces in the superior cavity as the articular disc is not bound tightly to the articular fossa. This movement, also known as translational movement, is the result of the mandible being in a forward position. Consequently, translational movement of the mandible takes place in the superior joint cavity between the mandibular fossa and the superior surface of the articular disc.

The condyle is forced more strongly against the disc and the disc against the fossa as muscle activity increases. This results in an increase in the interarticular pressure of these joint structures. In essence, the interarticular pressure is the pressure between the articular surfaces within the temporomandibular joint.

An increase in the interarticular pressure will result in the condyle positioning itself in the intermediate zone where the articular disc is the thinnest. On the other hand, as the interarticular pressure decreases and the disc space widens, this space is filled through the rotation of the articular disc to the anterior or posterior borders (Fig. **11**). The presence of interarticular pressure is vital as the articular surfaces will separate and the joint will technically dislocate when there is no interarticular pressure [75].

Furthermore, the width of the articular disc space varies with interarticular pressure. For example, when the mandible is at the closed rest position, the disc space widens as a result of the pressure being low. Conversely, the articular space narrows during clenching of the teeth due to the pressure being high.

It is also important to comprehend the relationship between the articular disc and the activity of the mandible. Whilst the condyle is in the closed joint position and the teeth are bought together, there is minimal elastic traction on the articular disc.

The force to retract the articular disc is increased during the opening movement of the mandible as the condyle is pulled forward along the articular eminence. This movement causes an increased stretching of the superior retrodiscal lamina. The superior retrodiscal lamina is also involved during the protrusive movement of the mandible. As the mandible is moved to and returned from a full forward position, the ligament will hold the articular disc rotated as far posteriorly on the condyle as allowed by the width of the articular space.

As mentioned previously, the muscles of mastication are composed of four pairs of muscles and one of those muscles is the lateral pterygoid muscle. During the closing movement of the mandible, the superior lateral pterygoid (Fig. **16**) is activated only in combination with the action of the elevator muscles [75]. This is also true during a power stroke.

In theory, it can be said that the superior lateral pterygoid is a protractor of the articular disc. As soon as the pterygoid muscle is active, the articular disc is pulled anteriorly and medially. Yet, this function does not take place during mandibular movements.

While observing the mechanics of chewing, it becomes obvious the significance of the purpose of the superior lateral pterygoid during the power stroke. The interarticular pressure on the biting side is reduced as soon as resistance is met such as when biting on hard food during the closing movement of the mandible. This occurs because of the force of closure being applied to food instead of the joint [75].

4.2. MASTICATION

By definition, mastication is the process of chewing food, in which the food is crushed and grounded against the maxillary and mandibular teeth. It is a complex function that utilizes the muscles of mastication, teeth and periodontal supportive structures and also the lips, cheeks, tongue, palate and salivary glands.

4.3. THE CHEWING STROKE

Mastication is composed of well-controlled and rhythmic parting and closure of the teeth in the maxilla and in the mandible. A chewing stroke is signified by every opening and closing of the mandible. A tear-shaped pattern can be used to describe the movement pattern of a complete chewing stroke. The entire movement can be separated into an opening phase and a closing phase. In addition, the closing movement can be further subdivided into the crushing phase and the grinding phase [75].

When the mandible is traced in the frontal plane during a single chewing stroke, the following sequence occurs:

1. During the opening phase, the mandible drops downward to a point where the incisal edges of the teeth are separated by a distance of 16 to 18 mm [78]. The mandible then moves in a lateral direction 5 to 6 mm from the midline. After this stage, the closing movement of the mandible begins.
2. The closing movement can be subdivided into two separate phases. The first phase is referred to as the crushing phase, where food is trapped during this stage between the maxillary and mandibular teeth. The second phase is known as the grinding phase. During this stage, the mandible is guided back to the intercuspal position by the occlusal surfaces of the teeth. Grinding and shearing of food mass are allowed by the passing of the cuspal inclines of the maxilla and mandibular teeth across each other.

During a regular chewing stroke, a small anterior movement of the mandible can be seen throughout the opening phase if the progress of a mandibular incisor is traced in the sagittal plane. On the contrary, the mandible follows a slightly posterior trace during the closing movement, concluding in an anterior movement returning to the starting maximum intercuspal location.

4.4. TOOTH CONTACTS DURING MASTICATION

It is important to gain an in-depth understanding into tooth contacts during mastication. Initially, only a small number of contacts occur between teeth when food is introduced into the oral cavity. The frequency of tooth contact increases as the food mass is broken down. Just before the food mass is swallowed, tooth contacts occur during every stroke in the final stages of mastication [79].

Accordingly, two types of tooth contact have been recognized [80]:

1. Gliding: during the opening and grinding phases of mastication, gliding occurs as the cuspal inclines pass by each other; and
2. Single: this takes place in the maximum intercuspal position.

During mastication, it has been observed that the average length of time for tooth contact is about 194 milliseconds [81]. Based on these observations, it can be said that the initial opening and final grinding phases of the chewing stroke are influenced or even dictated by these tooth contacts. Information related to the behavior of the chewing stroke based on the quantity as well as the quality of tooth contacts during mastication is conveyed constantly back to the central nervous system. The modification in the chewing stroke according to the type of food being chewed can then be made using this feedback mechanism.

4.5. FORCES OF MASTICATION

In general, the maximum biting force that can be applied to the teeth differs from individual to individual. In a previous study, it has been reported that females' maximum biting loads range from 35 to 44 kg, whereas males' biting loads vary from 53 to 64 kg [82]. It has also been demonstrated that individuals can increase their maximum biting force over a period of time through exercise and practice [82 - 84]. Furthermore, it has been suggested that the magnitude of the maximum biting force increases with age up to adolescence [84, 85].

Based on observation, the maximum amount of force that can be applied to a molar is normally several times higher than that can be applied to an incisor. Similarly, the amount of force placed in the region of the first molar is the greatest during chewing. Moreover, chewing mainly occurs around the second premolar and first molar when it comes to harder foods [75]. Consequently, an individual whose diet consists of high amounts of hard food will develop stronger biting force.

CHAPTER 5

Biomechanics of the Mandible

Abstract: The most frequently used biomechanical analogy for the mandible has been the Class III lever, in which the condyle acts as a fulcrum, the masticatory muscles as applied force, and the bite pressure as resistance. Various workers have suggested either directly or indirectly, that there is little or no reactive force at either mandibular condyle.

Mandibular movement occurs as a complex series of interrelated three-dimensional rotational and translational activities. Mandibular movement is limited by the ligaments and the articular surfaces of the temporomandibular joints as well as by the morphology and alignment of the teeth. The collective activities of masticatory muscles in different configurations have enabled us to perform a variety of mandibular movements.

Keywords: Biomechanics, Class III lever, Lever action, Mandibular movement, Non-lever action.

Undoubtedly, the Class III lever has been the most widely and frequently used biomechanical comparison for the human mandible (Fig. **17**), where the masticatory muscles such as the masseter and temporalis serve as the applied force, the bite force serve as resistance, and the condyle serve as a pivot point or fulcrum [86].

To achieve mechanical equilibrium, the Class III lever requires that the bite force be less than the applied force, so that the masticatory "machine" would have a mechanical advantage equal to less than one.

However, the hypothesis of the idea that the mandible behaves like a Class III lever has been disputed by researchers as they claimed that the articular fossa and the condyle are simply not designed by nature to endure the large resultant forces required by the lever model [87, 88]. In addition, criticisms were also raised by researchers due to the fact that the Class III lever model of the mandible does not take into consideration the issue regarding the center of mandibular rotation [88, 89].

Andy H. Choi and Besim Ben-Nissan

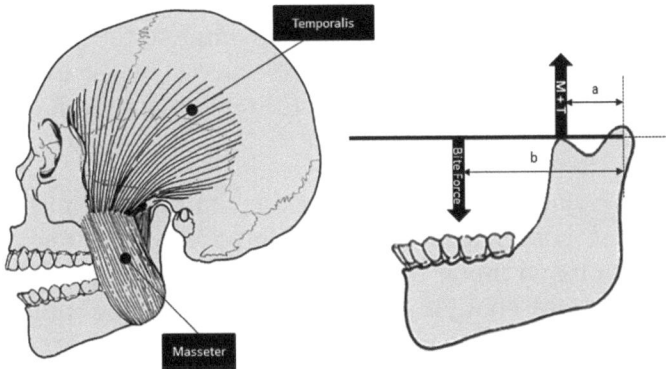

Fig. (17). The mandible as a Class III lever. The masseter and temporalis (M+T) as the applied force and the bite force as the resistance [86].

A concern was also discovered in two early studies relating to the idea of whether or not there is force at the condyle, instead of the condyle being a mechanism of force generation [88, 90]. A study by Roberts suggested that additional reaction force present at the condyle is not possible [90]. Since each force can be represented by a vector whose length is equal to the force magnitude, a closed triangle can be formed using vectors of the masseter and temporalis muscles along with the bite force. Furthermore, Roberts also argued that a triangle of these forces in equilibrium is entirely theoretical as complete and accurate data on the direction of the three forces and certainly on the magnitude of the masseter and temporalis muscle forces are not available [90]. Similarly, the absence of reaction forces at the condyle was also used as the basic assumption in a study by Roberts and Tattersall [88], in which they stated that no significant force is expended at the temporomandibular joint during elevation of the mandible.

Another approach that was used to investigate stresses of the mandible is to consider the mandible as a stationary beam. This method was first suggested by Parrington for analyzing external forces acting on the mandible during mastication [91]. This approach was later used by a number of researchers for examining the internal stresses and strains of mastication on the mandible [92 - 95].

It has been hypothesized that under conditions of equilibrium, the moments about any point will be equal to zero. For that reason, information about the amount of force that is being applied to the dentition will be the same as the value calculated from moments about the instantaneous center of rotation, the center of the mandibular condyle and the center of the chin or any other point in space [96].

Despite the fact that examining the mandibles of mammals purely in the lateral projection is perhaps suitable for incisor or bilateral molar biting, a study by Hylander suggested that such an analysis is incomplete for unilateral biting [97]. This is because the projected bite point is never actually located in the mid-sagittal plane. Consequently, it is also useful to analyze the human mandible in the frontal projection.

In his later study, Hylander concluded that the contralateral mandibular condyle could have a large compressive reaction force acting across it during both unilateral mastication and molar biting, while lower levels of compressive stress act across the ipsilateral condyle during mastication. In some instances during unilateral molar biting, the ipsilateral condyle might even be free of stress, or there may be tensile stress acting across it [98].

In addition, it has also been suggested that widening or narrowing of the dental arches may instead only change the proportion of the force that each condyle will sustain but not the total magnitude of force at the condyles. The nature of muscle positions in the sagittal plane dictates that condylar forces will occur [97, 99].

5.1. NON-LEVER ACTION HYPOTHESES

Arguments also exist concerning the validity of the lever hypothesis and the human mandible behaving as a Class III lever. A number of researchers, have either indirectly or directly, suggested that there is little or no reactive force at either mandibular condyle.

In the 1920s, Wilson was one of the first researchers to disagree with the lever action hypothesis of human jaw mechanics. Wilson argues that since the resultant force of the temporalis, masseter, and medial pterygoid muscles lies perpendicular to the occlusal plane, there can be no reaction force at the mandibular condyle. For that reason, it was incorrect to view the human mandible as a lever [100].

Another researcher who advanced the non-lever theory of mandible mechanics was Robinson [87]. According to Robinson, the resultant adductor muscle force passes through the first molar tooth. Assuming that the resultant force has been correctly determined, biting on the first molar in this projection would indeed result in a non-lever action of the mandible and that all the resultant muscle force would be transmitted directly through the teeth.

A study by Frank has also supported the notion of the non-lever action of the mandible [101]. The arguments put forward by Frank were based on the radiographic examinations of the human mandibular condyle. In each of the radiographs, Frank noticed that the condyle was never in direct contact with the articular eminence. Based on these findings, Frank concluded that the mandible could not function as a lever because the condyle was not functioning as a fulcrum.

Another worker to suggest non-lever action in the human mandible was Gingerich [102]. Gingerich established that the mandible is functioning as a link between the adductor muscle force and the bite force instead of a lever during biting. This opinion was later supported by Tattersall, who also suggested that the mandible does not function as a lever during chewing or biting [103].

5.2. MANDIBULAR MOVEMENT

Mandibular movement occurs as a complex series of interrelated three-dimensional rotational and translational activities. Mandibular movement is limited by the ligaments and the articular surfaces of the temporomandibular joints as well as by the morphology and alignment of the teeth.

The collective activities of masticatory muscles in different configurations have enabled us to perform a variety of mandibular movements. It is especially important to realize that one muscle may act synergistically with different muscles at different times. In no instance does a muscle act as an independent unit. Instead, muscles act in large groups.

As mentioned earlier, the most important muscles that affect movements of the mandible can be divided into three major groups:

1. Elevators: the temporalis, masseter and medial pterygoid muscles;
2. Depressors: the digastrics; and
3. Protractors: the lateral pterygoid muscles.

5.2.1. Mandibular Rest Position

It is commonly assumed that the mandible is maintained in a relatively constant position in relation to the maxilla when a person is relaxed, and that the maintenance of this position is the function of some postural control mechanism that produces a low level of activity in the elevator muscles to oppose the effects of gravity [104].

Hypothetically, it is possible to record the electromyographic (EMG) activity of the elevator muscles if they were actively engaged in maintaining the position of the mandible against gravity in the rest position. A number of studies have reported low levels of activity in the masseter, temporalis, lateral pterygoid and suprahyoid muscles at rest [105 - 109].

Furthermore, a study has discovered there are changes in the activity of these muscles when the body is tilted, suggesting that the resting activity may be adjusted according to gravitational effects [108].

5.2.2. Opening Movement

During simple opening movement of the mandible (Fig. **18**), the mandible rotates around a frontal axis that passes approximately through the centers of the two condyles while the axis itself progresses in space [110].

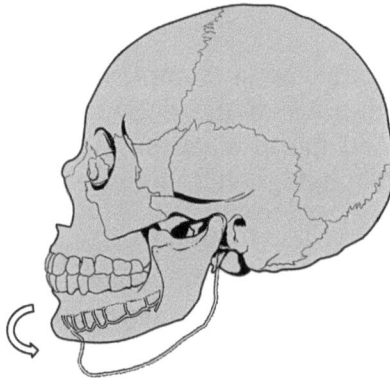

Fig. (18). Opening movement of the mandible.

In his EMG analysis of temporomandibular movement, Moyers postulated that the opening movement is the result of the combined actions of the digastric and lateral pterygoid muscles [111]. If this movement occurs without resistance, the depressors act without any great force.

According to studies by Sicher and Du Brul [112] and Hylander [97], the condyles rotate against the articular disc around a transverse axis as they slide downward and forward along the posterior slope of the articular eminence during the opening movement of the mandible. The movement is influenced by an initial activity of the lateral pterygoids, which first fix the condyles firmly against the posterior slope of the eminence. This is immediately followed by contraction of the digastric muscles, and the sustained activity of both muscle pairs acting as a force-couple. This motion affects all the other muscles anchored to the mandible, but it also has a receding influence on muscles more peripheral to the central action. Thus, the elevators of the jaw must lengthen to act as mild balancers and to ensure the opening movement is carried out smoothly.

5.2.3. Protrusive Mandibular Movement

A protrusive mandibular movement occurs when the mandible moves forward from the centric occlusion position. Any area of a tooth that contacts an opposing tooth during protrusive movement is considered as protrusive contact (Fig. **19**).

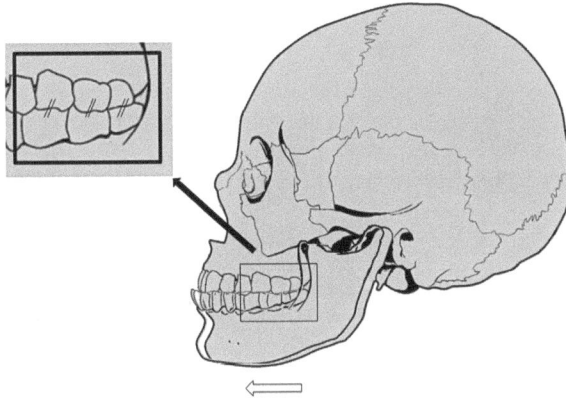

Fig. (19). Protrusion of the mandible.

A number of studies have shown that forward thrust of the mandible is the result of contraction of the inferior head of the lateral pterygoid muscles and holding action of the masseter and medial pterygoid muscle [111, 113, 114]. The temporalis muscle is not active during this movement, and the depressors are only active to a minor degree.

5.2.4. Laterotrusive Mandibular Movement

During a lateral mandibular movement, the right and left mandibular posterior teeth move across their opposing teeth in different directions. If the mandible moves laterally to the left (Fig. **20**), the left mandibular posterior teeth will move laterally across their opposing teeth. However, the right mandibular posterior teeth will move medially across their opposing teeth. The potential contact areas for these teeth are in different locations and are therefore designated by different names.

According to a previous study [112], one condyle and disc slide downward, medially and forward along the articular eminence while the other rotates laterally around a vertical axis during the lateral movement. The lateral pterygoid muscle, inserted on the inwardly thrust medial pole of the condyle, pulls inward and forward in the horizontal plane. The horizontal fibers of the temporalis muscle inserted at the posterior tip of the coronoid process pull outward and backward. These muscles, operating as a force-couple, contribute to the torque of the rotating condyle necessary to effect chewing on this side.

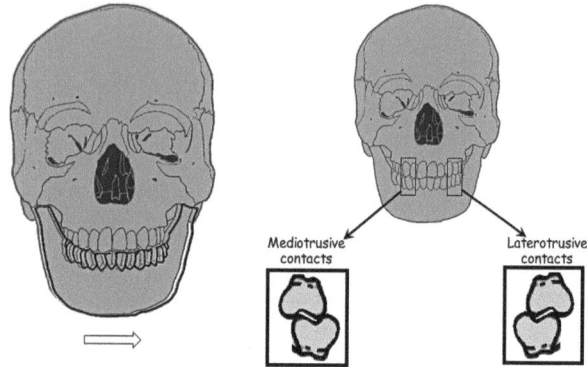

Fig. (20). Left laterotrusive movement of the mandible [75].

5.2.5. Retrusive Mandibular Movement

A retrusive movement occurs when the mandible shifts posteriorly from centric occlusion (Fig. **21**). During a retrusive movement, the mandibular buccal cusps move distally across the occlusal surface of their opposing maxillary teeth. Retrusive contacts occur on the reverse inclines of the protrusive contacts since the movement is exactly opposite.

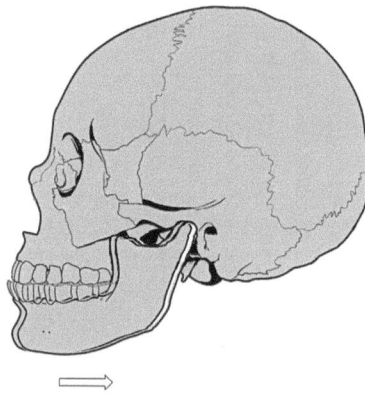

Fig. (21). Retrusive movement of the mandible [75].

In the retracting movement, the middle and posterior fibers of the temporalis muscle combine forces with the depressors, while the remaining elevators exhibit varying amounts of activity [113].

5.2.6. Closing Movement

The elevators of the mandible execute the closing movement, which returns the jaw to the rest or occlusal position (Fig. **22**). If the mouth is opened to its maximal extent, the timing of the activation and relaxation of the different parts of these muscles is important for proper closure.

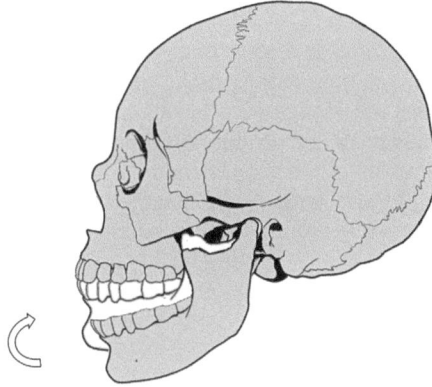

Fig. (22). Closing movement of the mandible.

CHAPTER 6

Mathematical Analysis of the Mandible

Abstract: Numerous muscles acting simultaneously on the mandible are utilized to create a bite force. Defining the involvement of each muscle to the creation of this bite force is the biggest challenge as it cannot be resolved using the conditions of static equilibrium. Estimation of the temporomandibular joint (TMJ) forces from mathematical models has a long history but has led to conflicting results. The biggest disagreement has been over whether the TMJ is even load bearing. To model completely all of the forces involved in the production of the TMJ reaction force will be difficult as all force vectors need to be established in three-dimensions. Three different approaches have been proposed to calculate all the muscle forces and the forces in the temporomandibular joints during biting.

Keywords: Barbenel, Bite force, Muscle tension, Physiological cross-sectional areas, Pruim, Temporomandibular joint forces, Throckmorton.

As mentioned earlier, numerous muscles acting simultaneously on the mandible are utilized to create a bite force. Defining the involvement of each muscle to the creation of this bite force is the biggest challenge as it cannot be resolved using the conditions of static equilibrium.

Postulating that each muscle produces a force relative to its cross-sectional area is one simple answer which has been proposed [115]. For the temporomandibular joint (TMJ), the unknowns for bilateral static bite force would then be the magnitude of the proportionality constant along with the direction and magnitude of the reaction force at the temporomandibular joint. A study by Throckmorton and Throckmorton suggested that these could be ascertained by projecting and balancing the vertical and horizontal force components onto the sagittal plane and the moments around an axis perpendicular to the sagittal plane [116].

Approximation of the TMJ forces using mathematical models has a long history but has led to contradictory outcomes. The biggest disagreement has been over whether the TMJ is even load bearing as previously discussed [86 - 88, 90, 97, 98, 100, 102, 117 - 122]. To model completely all of the forces involved in the production of the TMJ reaction force will be difficult as all force vectors need to

Andy H. Choi and Besim Ben-Nissan

be established in three-dimensions. Calculation of the total joint reaction force requires:

1. The direction, magnitude, and moment arm lengths of each muscle force; and
2. The direction and magnitude of the bite force.

The direction and extent of the bite force can be quickly evaluated using force transducers, while the moment arm lengths can be determined from lateral cephalograms of human subjects [122].

The force a muscle can apply is not only governed by physiological parameters (such as the muscle length, speed of contraction, and level of neuronal activation) but also by anatomical parameters, such as the total cross-section of all muscle fibers, referred to as physiological cross-section [123, 124]. Data on the physiological cross-sectional areas can be used to determine the forces of the various muscles (Table **6**). The value of maximum muscle tension (Γ), a relationship between the maximum force exerted by a muscle and its physiological cross-sectional area, is shown in Table **7**.

Table 6. Physiological cross-sectional areas (cm^2) of the muscles of mastication [123, 124].

Muscles	Schumacher	Pruim *et al.*
Medial Pterygoid	1.97	5.3[a]
Masseter	3.02	
Temporalis	3.81	4.2[b]
Openers	-----	1.0[c]
Lateral Pterygoid	1.83	2.1
[a] Includes medial pterygoid and masseter		
[b] Includes anterior and posterior temporalis		
[c] Only digastric was measured		

Table 7. Average maximum muscle tension (Γ) in N/m^2 [105, 106, 124 - 128].

Investigators	Maximum Muscle Tension (Γ)
Fick	1.0×10^6
Morris	0.9×10^6
Carlsoo	1.1×10^6
Hettinger	0.4×10^6
Ikai and Fukunaga	0.7×10^6
Pruim *et al.*	1.4×10^6

Two methods have been employed to determine the magnitudes of the muscle forces. In the first method, researchers attempted to approximate the force generated by each muscle from the total cross-sectional area of the muscle [117, 123,124, 129, 130]. In the second method, the integrated electromyogram (iEMG) from each muscle was used as an estimate of muscle force [121, 124, 131] (Table **8**).

Table 8. Averaged calculated maximum muscle forces (N) in each single muscle group and related standard deviations [105, 106, 123, 124, 130, 132].

Muscle	Carlsoo	Schumacher	Pruim *et al.*	Osborn and Baragar
Medial Pterygoid	299 ± 46	190	639 ± 176[b]	254
Masseter	614 ± 107	340		450
Anterior Temporalis	519 ± 102	420[a]	362 ± 65	264
Posterior Temporalis	305 ± 102		197 ± 26	323
Openers	------	-----	115 ± 40	107
Lateral Pterygoid	525	175	378 ± 106	382
[a] Anterior Temporalis + Posterior Temporalis				
[b] Medial Pterygoid + Masseter				

6.1. ANALYSIS BY BARBENEL

Barbenel [120] presented the first analysis of the force actions at the TMJ. The co-ordinate system used in the analysis is presented in Fig. (**23**).

During biting, the force system imposed on the mandible from a stationary position is composed of three different forces:

1. Forces due to muscle action;
2. Forces due to occlusal load; and
3. The force at the TMJ.

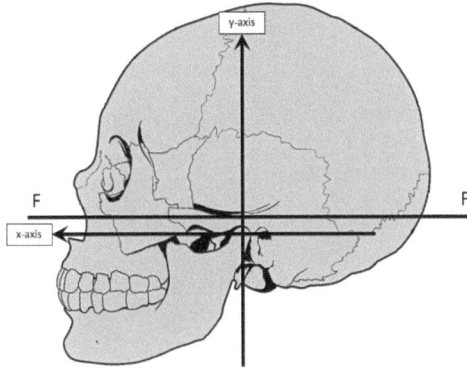

Fig. (23). Co-ordinate axes used in joint force analysis. The z-axis is directed inwards along the intercondylar axis [120].

6.1.1. Forces Due to Muscle Action

The analyses were centered on the mandible in the rest position, with the muscles of each side acting evenly. In the analysis, the muscle forces used were those produced by the masseter (F_{mass}), the temporalis (F_{temp}), the internal pterygoid (F_{int}), and the external pterygoid (F_{ext}) muscles (Fig. **24**).

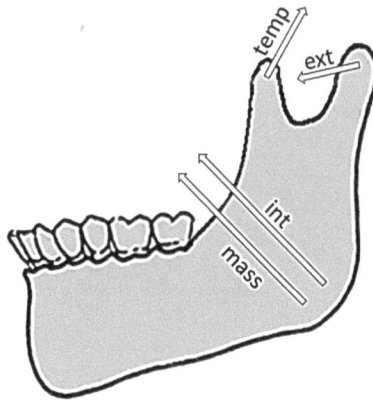

Fig. (24). Muscles considered in the analysis [120].

6.1.2. Forces Due to Occlusal Load

This load was arbitraries considered acting equally on each side of the mandible, with a magnitude of L and directed at an angle θ to the y-axis (Fig. **25**).

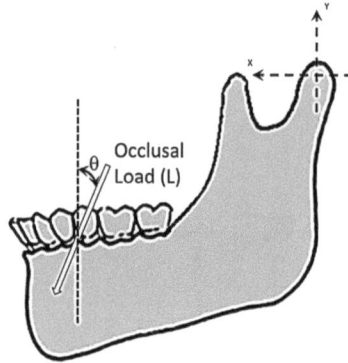

Fig. (25). Occlusal load parameter [120].

The moment of the load about the intercondylar axis:

$$L \left(X \cos \theta - Y \sin \theta \right) \tag{1}$$

where X and Y is the co-ordinate of the point at which the line of action of the load intersects the occlusal plane.

6.1.3. The Force at the TMJ

This force was assumed to have magnitude R and to act at an angle of ϕ to the y-axis (Fig. **26**).

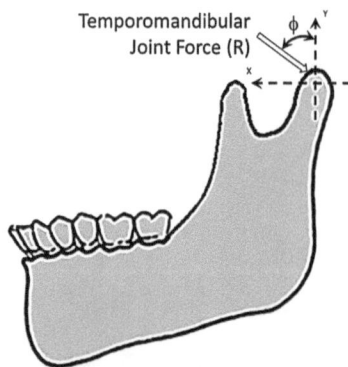

Fig. (26). Temporomandibular joint force parameter [120].

Taking moments about the intercondylar axis and utilizing the determined muscle force components (Table **9**), three equations of equilibrium for the mandible subjected to the force system are obtained:

- Force component in the x-direction is equal to zero:

$$0.84F_{mass} + 0.84F_{temp} + 0.77F_{int} - 0.17F_{ext} - R\cos\phi - L\cos\theta = 0 \qquad (2)$$

- Force component in the y-direction is equal to zero:

$$0.55F_{mass} - 0.46F_{temp} + 0.50F_{int} + 0.91F_{ext} - R\sin\phi - L\sin\theta = 0 \qquad (3)$$

- Sum of the moments of the forces about any axis is equal to zero:

$$2.7F_{mass} + 2.6F_{temp} + 2.3F_{int} - L(X\cos\theta - Y\sin\theta) = 0 \qquad (4)$$

Table 9. Values of mean and standard error in the mean of muscle force parameters [120].

Muscle	Force Component			Moment Arm about Intercondylar Axis (cm)
	x	y	z	
Masseter	0.55	0.84	-0.12	2.7
Temporalis	-0.46	0.84	-0.18	2.6
Internal Pterygoid	0.50	0.78	0.38	2.3
External Pterygoid	0.91	-0.17	0.39	0.0

6.2. ANALYSIS BY PRUIM, DE JONGH, TEN BOSCH

In the 1980s, Pruim and co-workers have chosen a mechanical approach to estimate all muscle forces and the forces in the TMJs during bilateral biting at three separate locations on the human dentition [124]. The centroids of the mandibular condyles were chosen as the origins of an x- and y-axis system. The x-axis was oriented parallel to the mandibular occlusal plane, thus to the bite plane in the experimental set-up (Fig. **27**).

In order to determine these forces, a calculation program was used and fed with data on bilaterally measured bite forces and iEMG activity in the principal muscles.

Bite forces were measured bilaterally using two calibrated steel transducers provided with strain gauges. Surface electrodes were utilized bilaterally to measure the electromyographic activity in the main muscles. However, the activity in the lateral pterygoid muscles was not recorded.

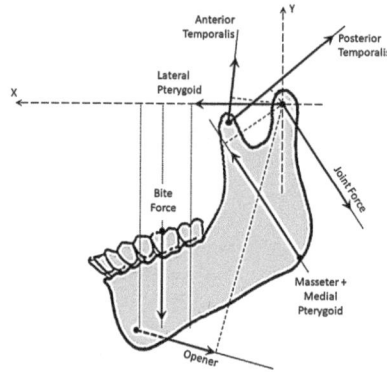

Fig. (27). Mathematical model based on the mandible [124].

Several assumptions were necessary:

1. Forces exerted by contracting muscles can be represented by vectors.
2. Direction of these vectors can be described by connecting lines from the centroids of the origins and the insertions of the muscles.
3. Forces of the masseter and medial pterygoid muscles can be signified by a single vector. The lateral pterygoid muscle acts in a direction parallel to the occlusal plane; consequently, the force the lateral pterygoid muscle produced contains no y-component.
4. The EMG-activity of the masseter muscle is also illustrative for the medial pterygoid muscle. The activity in the floor of the mouth is representative for the mouth openers.

For each experimental subject, there exists a muscle independent value Γ (in N/m^2), which relates the maximum force exerted by a muscle ($F_{m(max)}$) to its physiological cross-section ϕ_m (in m^2) (eq. (5)).

$$F_{m(max)} = \Gamma \cdot \phi_m \qquad (5)$$

The values of the physiological cross-section, as determined by Schumacher [123] for males correspond to the values for test subjects (Table **6**).

The muscle force exerted during isometric contraction (F_m) is directly proportional to the iEMG. The relationship between the iEMG and muscle force can then be expressed as follows:

$$F_m = \left(\frac{iEMG_{m(actual)}}{iEMG_{m(max)}} \right) F_{m(max)} \qquad (6)$$

where $iEMG_{m(max)}$ is the maximum value of $iEMG_m$ of a single muscle ever recorded during a complete experimental session from a pair of electrode.

The laws of static equilibrium are used in calculating all forces:

- The sum of the moments = 0

$$\sum F_m a_m + F_b a_b = 0 \qquad (7)$$

where F_m is the muscle force exerted during isometric contraction; F_b is the sum of both left and right bite forces; a_m is the muscle lever arm; and a_b is the bite force lever arm.

- When the moments are referred to the origin and eq. (6) is used, this leads to:

$$\sum_{muscles} \left(\frac{iEMG_{m(actual)}}{iEMG_{m(max)}} \right) \Gamma \phi_m a_m + F_b a_b = 0 \qquad (8)$$

iEMG$_m$ values and sum of both bite force were measured in each bite, the arms were obtained from the cephalometric data. Using the values of physiological cross-sections of muscle (ϕ) from Table **6**, Γ was calculated from eq. (8) for each bite.

After substituting of Γ in eq. (5), all forces in the elevator and antagonistic muscles during that bite were calculated.

- The sum of the x-component = 0

$$\sum_{muscles} F_m \cos \alpha_m + F_j \cos \alpha_j + F_p = 0 \qquad (9)$$

- The sum of the y-component = 0

$$\sum_{muscles} F_m \sin \alpha_m + F_j \sin \alpha_j - F_b = 0 \qquad (10)$$

6.3. ANALYSIS BY THROCKMORTON AND THROCKMORTON

A two-dimensional model (Fig. **28**) is used to evaluate the magnitude (F_{TMJ}) and direction (ϕ) of the total joint reaction force [116].

The direction and extent of the TMJ reaction force are determined using the laws of statics in two stages. In static equilibrium, the sum of all moments is zero and the sum of all forces is zero.

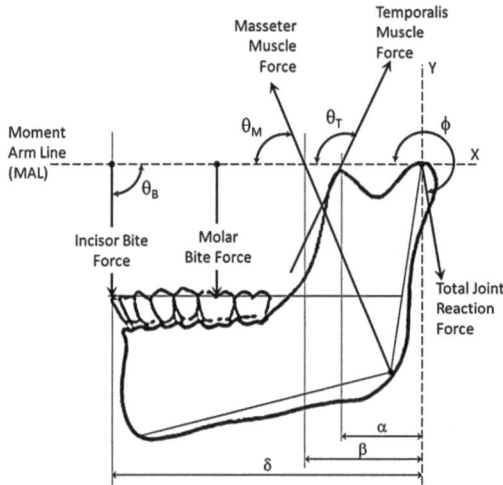

Fig. (28). Diagrammatic representation of the two-dimensional model used to calculate total joint reaction force [116]. θ_T is the angle with the occlusal plane of temporalis muscle force; θ_M is the angle with the occlusal plane of masseter muscle force; θ_B is the angles with the occlusal plane of the bite forces; α is the moment arm for temporalis muscle force; β is the moment arm for masseter muscle force; δ is the moment arm for the bite force; and ϕ is the angle of the total joint reaction force with the moment arm line (MAL).

The first step is to calculate the magnitude of the muscle forces from the sum of the moments:

$$F_{temp}\, \alpha + F_{mass}\, \beta + F_{bite}\, \delta = 0 \qquad (11)$$

where F_{temp}, F_{mass}, and F_{bite} are the forces exerted by the temporalis, masseter, and bite force, respectively (Fig. **28**).

The most widely used approach for evaluating the moment of the jaw muscles is to determine the perpendicular distance between the muscle vector and the center of joint rotation. The product of this distance (moment arm length) and the extent of the muscle force vector is the moment of that muscle.

Another approach is to divide each muscle force into components that are parallel and perpendicular to a line parallel to the occlusal plane and passing through the center of joint rotation. This line is the moment arm line. Only components of force that are perpendicular to the moment arm line produce a moment and the length of the moment arm is the distance from the center of joint rotation to the muscle vector (Fig. **28**).

Eq. (11) can then be further expanded:

$$F_{temp} \sin \theta_T \, \alpha + F_{mass} \sin \theta_M \, \beta + F_{bite} \sin \theta_B \, \delta = 0 \qquad \text{(12)}$$

Despite the fact that the magnitude of the two muscle forces (masseter and temporalis) are not directly measurable, the magnitude of one muscle force can be conveyed in terms of the other if the relative magnitudes of the muscle forces are estimated:

$$F_{mass} = K F_{temp} \qquad \text{(13)}$$

where K is a proportionality constant between the two muscle forces.

By substituting the relative muscle forces into eq. (12), the magnitudes of the muscle forces (masseter and temporalis) can now be solved:

$$F_{mass} = \left[\frac{F_{bite} \sin \theta_B \, \delta}{K \sin \theta_T \, \alpha + \sin \theta_M \, \beta} \right] \qquad \text{(14)}$$

Finally, the value of F_{temp} can be determined from eq. (13).

Using the sum of forces, the temporomandibular joint reaction force (F_{TMJ}) can be solved once the magnitude of each muscle force is determined:

$$F_{mass} + F_{temp} - F_{bite} - F_{TMJ} = 0 \qquad \text{(15)}$$

Each force is divided into vertical components of force which are perpendicular to the moment arm line, and horizontal components of force that are parallel to the moment arm line.

The vertical components of force produce rotation and the horizontal components of force produce translation [133].

- For the vertical component of the joint reaction forces (FJV):

$$FJV = F_{mass} \sin \theta_M + F_{temp} \sin \theta_T - F_{bite} \sin \theta_B \qquad \textbf{(16)}$$

- For the horizontal component of the joint reaction forces (FJH):

$$FJH = F_{mass} \cos \theta_M + F_{temp} \cos \theta_T - F_{bite} \cos \theta_B \qquad \textbf{(17)}$$

- Total joint reaction force, and its direction ϕ:

$$F_{TMJ} = \sqrt{FJV^2 + FJH^2} \qquad \textbf{(18)}$$

$$\phi = Arc \sin \frac{FJV}{F_{TMJ}} \qquad \textbf{(19)}$$

CHAPTER 7

Finite Element Method

Abstract: The finite element method is a mathematical approach used to examine continua and structures. Typically, the problem at hand is too difficult to be resolved in a satisfactory manner using classical analytical means. Introduced initially as an approach used to explain structural mechanics problems, finite element analysis was rapidly acknowledged as a universal technique of mathematical approximation to all physical problems that can be modelled by a differential equation description. The application of finite element analysis in dentistry related to the deformations during functional loadings and in the design and analysis of implants accelerated after the 1980's. This method has been widely accepted and applied in engineering and biomedical systems with increasing frequency for stress analyses of soft and hard tissues, bone and bone-prosthesis structures, fracture fixation devices, and dental implants and devices ever since. The finite element approach has also been applied in nanomechanical testing and nanoindentation to assess the biomechanical properties of nanocoatings on implants and devices.

Keywords: Anisotropic, Convergence test, Elastic modulus, Element characteristic matrix, Finite element analysis, Finite element modeling, Isotropic, Material properties, Non-linear analysis, Poisson's ratio, Transversely isotropic.

Introduced initially as an approach used to explain structural mechanics problems, finite element analysis was rapidly acknowledged as a universal technique of mathematical approximation to all physical problems that can be modelled by a differential equation description. The problem may concern stress analysis, heat conduction, or any of several other areas.

7.1. SUMMARY OF FINITE ELEMENT HISTORY

Beginning in 1906, researchers proposed a "lattice analogy" aimed at stress analysis. The continuum was substituted by a methodical pattern of elastic bars. Properties of the bars were selected in a way that caused displacements of the joints to approximate displacements of points in the continuum. The method sought to capitalize on well-known methods of structural analysis.

Andy H. Choi and Besim Ben-Nissan

A German American mathematician by the name of Richard L. Courant emerges as the first to suggest the finite element method (FEM) as we know it today [134]. In a 1941 mathematics lecture, which was later published in 1943, piecewise polynomial interpolation over triangular subregions and the principle of stationary potential energy was applied by him to examine the Saint-Venant torsion problem. Courant's work was ignored until it was later further expanded by engineers independently [135].

At the time, none of the abovementioned work was of much practical value as computer power was not available to create and resolve large series of simultaneous algebraic equations. It is not accidental that the expansion of finite element analysis overlapped with major advances in programming language and digital computers.

By 1953, engineers had created and determined stiffness equations in matrix format using digital computers. A vast amount of this work was carried out within the aerospace sector. A large finite element problem during that time contained a hundred degrees of freedom. Turner, at the Boeing Airplane Company in 1953, proposed that a triangular plane stress element could be employed to model the skin of a delta wing. Published almost simultaneously with similar work carried out in England, this work signifies the commencement of the widespread application of finite elements. Much of this early work went unrecognized as a result of company policies against publication [136 - 138].

The term "finite element method" was devised in 1960 by Clough. The practical value of the method was becoming clear. New elements intended for stress analysis purposes were created, mostly by physical argument and intuition. FEM gained respectability in 1963 when it was acknowledged as having a sound numerical foundation; it can be thought of as the explanation of a variational problem by minimization of a functional. Consequently, the method was being applied to all field problems which can be modeled in a variational form [139, 140].

During the late 1960s and early 1970s, large general-purpose finite element computer programs emerged and examples of such programs include ANSYS, ASKA and NASTRAN. Each of these programs contained numerous forms of elements and could perform dynamic, static, and heat transfer investigation. Extra capabilities were quickly incorporated. In addition, pre-processors (for data input) and post-processors (for result evaluation) were also included. These processors depend on graphics and make it easier, cheaper, and quicker to perform finite element analysis. Graphics development became intensive during the early 1980s as hardware and software for interactive graphics became accessible and affordable.

Normally, a general-purpose finite element program contains over 100,000 lines of code and usually resides on a mainframe or a superminicomputer. However, during the mid-1980s, adaptations of general-purpose programs started to appear on personal computers. Hundreds of analysis and analysis-related programs are now available, large or small, general or narrow, cheap or expensive, for lease or for purchase.

Today, finite element is also used to routinely solve problems for heat transfer, fluid flow, lubrication, electric and magnetic fields, and many other problems that were previously intractable. Finite element analysis is used in the designing of buildings, electric motors, heat engines, ships, airframes and spacecraft.

Since the beginning of the 1970, finite element analysis has been used extensively in orthopedic biomechanics to determine stresses in human bones during functional loadings. The application of finite element analysis in dentistry related to the deformations during functional loadings and in the design and analysis of implants accelerated after the 1980's.

Later, this method has been widely accepted and applied in engineering and biomedical systems with increasing frequency for stress analyses of soft and hard tissues, bone and bone-prosthesis structures, fracture fixation devices, and dental implants and devices.

The finite element approach has also been applied in nanomechanical testing and nanoindentation to assess the biomechanical properties of nanocoatings on metallic implants and devices.

7.2. THE BASICS

The finite element method is a mathematical approach used to examine continua and structures. Typically, the problem at hand is too difficult to be resolved in a satisfactory manner using classical analytical means.

The finite element process generates a lot of simultaneous algebraic equations, which are created and calculated on a digital computer. Finite element calculations are carried out on laptops, mainframes, and personal computers. Results are seldom precise. However, errors are reduced by processing more equations, and results accurate enough for engineering applications are attainable at reasonable costs.

Finite element analysis examines a complex problem by redefining it as the summation of the solutions of a series of interrelated simpler problems. The first stage involves subdividing (that is, discretize) the complex geometry into a suitable set of smaller "elements" of "finite" dimensions. This forms the "mesh" model of the investigated structure when combined (Fig. **29**).

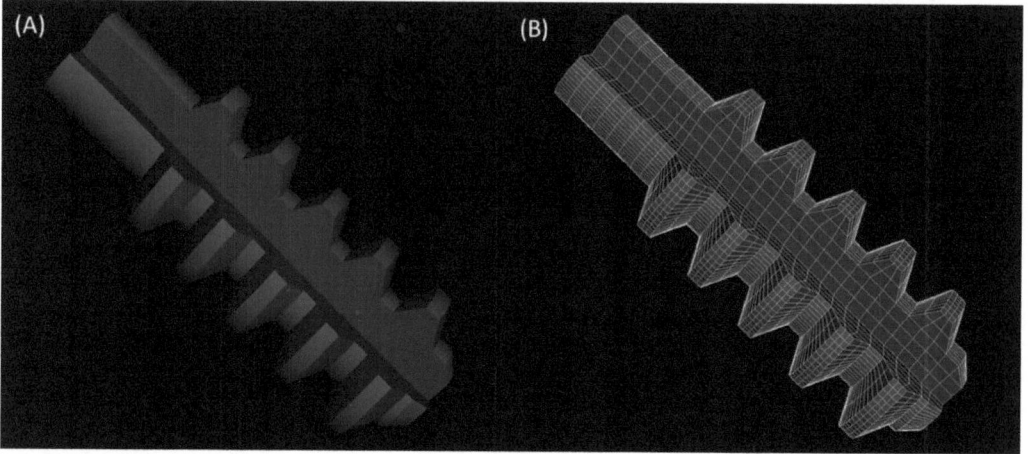

Fig. (29). Schematic illustration of a dental implant. (**A**) Solid model; (**B**) Finite element mesh.

Each element can undertake a specific geometric shape (that is, square, cube, triangle, tetrahedron, for example) with a specific internal strain function. The equilibrium equations between the displacements taking place at its corner points or "nodes" and the external forces acting on the element can be written using these functions, the actual geometry of the element, and a suite of boundary conditions such as constrain points. One equation for each degree of freedom will be created for each node of the element. In general, these equations are appropriately written in matrix form for utilization in a computer algorithm.

From the above example, and as a whole, the finite element method models a structure as an assembly of small parts (elements). A simple geometry is used to define each element and therefore is much easier to examine than the actual structure. In essence, the finite element approach approximates a complicated solution by a model that consists of piecewise-continuous simple solutions. Elements are called "finite" to separate them from differential elements used in calculus.

7.3. GENERAL PRINCIPLES

The finite element method is a method of piecewise calculation where the approximating function ϕ is created by linking simple functions, each defined over a small region (element). A finite element is a region in space in which a function ϕ is introduced from nodal values of ϕ on the boundary of the region in such a manner that interelement continuity of φ tends to be preserved in the assembly.

Typically, a finite element analysis consists of the following stages. Decisions by the analyst and provision of input data for the computer program are required during steps 1, 4, and 5. Steps 2, 3, 6, and 7 are carried out automatically by the computer program.

1. Divide the continuum or structure into finite elements. Mesh generation programs referred to as pre-processors assist the user in doing this work.
2. Devise the properties of each element. In stress analysis, nodal loads connected to all element deformation states that are allowed are determined. In heat transfer, nodal heat fluxes related with all element temperature fields that are allowed are defined.
3. Assemble elements to construct the finite element model of the structure.
4. Apply the known loads. In stress analysis: nodal forces and/or moments. In heat transfer: nodal heat fluxes.
5. In stress analysis, indicate how the structure is supported. This stage requires the calibration of numerous nodal displacement to known values, typically zero. In heat transfer, impose all known values of nodal temperature in which certain temperatures are usually known.
6. Solve simultaneous linear algebraic equations to ascertain nodal degrees of freedom. In stress analysis, this means nodal displacements. In heat transfer, this means nodal temperatures.
7. In stress analysis, calculate element strains from the nodal degrees of freedom and the element displacement field interpolation, and ultimately determine stresses from strains. In heat transfer, calculate element heat fluxed from the nodal temperatures and the element temperature field interpolation. Output interpretation programs, referred to as post-processors, assist the analyst organize the output and display it in graphical form.

7.4. MODEL CONSTRUCTION

The projected response of the finite model is dependent on the appropriate choice of the type of elements and thus achieving the objectives set out for the analysis, i.e. stress analysis, heat transfer. As a result, FEA offers a wide diversity of different element types, which can be classified according to family, order and topology.

The element family defines the attributes of displacement and geometry which the element is aiming to model. Typically for structural models, the most widely used families include one-dimensional (1-D) beam elements, two-dimensional (2-D) plane stress and plane strain elements, axisymmetric elements, and three-dimensional (3-D) shell and solid elements (Fig. **30**).

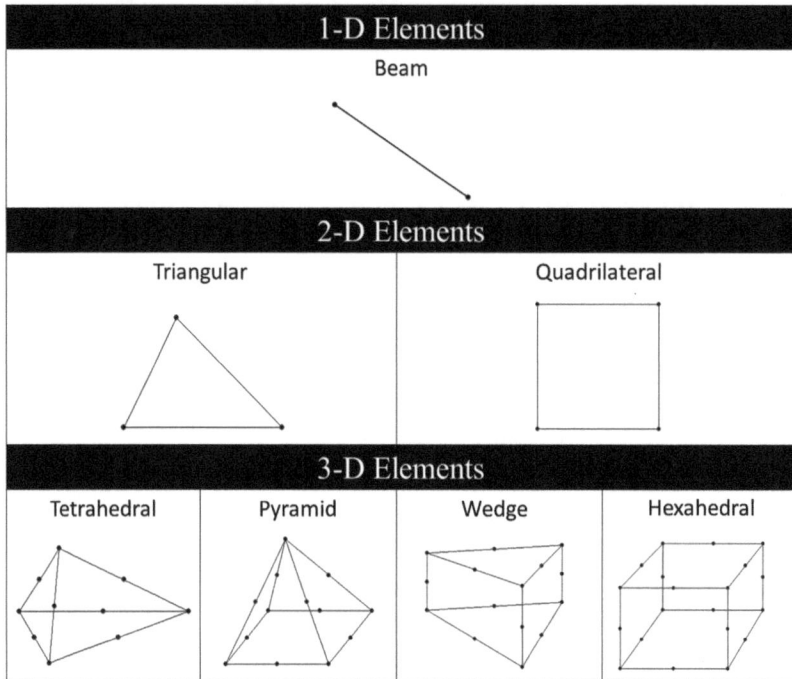

Fig. (30). Types of elements used in finite element analysis.

In terms of modeling beam-like structures where the bending moments and overall deflection can be predicted and where the length is much greater than other dimensions, the use of beam elements are advantageous. This type of model on the other hand will not determine the local stress concentrations at joints or at points where load is applied. Plane stress elements are ideal for thin 2-D structures, where stresses out of the plane can be ignored. Plane strain elements simulate a special 3-D stress state, occurring when out-of-plane deformation is constrained (for example, in relatively thick plates).

By utilizing well-defined characteristics of an axisymmetric geometry, 3-D stress fields can be modelled and simulated under 2-D conditions through the use of axisymmetrical elements. Shell elements can be applied effectively for 3-D structures which are thin in comparison to all other dimensions, for instance sheet metal parts where bending and in-plane forces are vital. On the other hand, these elements as a consequence of local bending effects will not predict stresses which vary throughout the thickness of the shell. All 3-D conditions are preferably modeled using solid elements. Yet, the order of magnitude of such a solid model may impose practical limits on the choice of those elements given that the computational effort of most finite element solvers is roughly proportional to the number of equations and the square of the bandwidth. Therefore, in each finite element model and analysis, an acceptable reduction of a 3-D situation should be seriously considered.

Elements can also be classified according to order. Linear elements possess two nodes along each edge, while parabolic have three. Compared to lower-order elements, higher-order elements are less stiff, and this is related to bending since extra nodes provide more degrees of freedom. A degree of freedom signifies the freedom of movement (rotational or translator) for a particular node in space. For example, six degrees of freedom are found at each of the unrestrained nodes for shell elements: three rotations around the x, y, and z-axes and three translations (x, y, and z). Conversely, the unrestrained nodes in 2-D elements only have two translational degrees of freedom, while 3-D (solid) elements only have three. An increase in the number of degrees of freedom creates more variables in the stiffness formulation, which is more computer-intensive. For an equal mesh grid, higher-order elements can provide results that are more accurate, but a finer grid of lower-order elements can turn out to be more efficient with the same accuracy.

Element topology implies to the general shape of the element, i.e. triangular or quadrilateral (Fig. **30**). The topology also depends on the family of the element, such as 2-D or 3-D. Typically, in complex structural models, quadrilateral elements may be thought of as more ideal than triangular elements as quadrilaterals can match the true displacement with more accuracy attributable to a higher number of degrees of freedom. In addition, the number of elements in meshes constructed using triangular elements normally is higher. On the other hand, the simplicity of triangular elements makes them very attractive, for instance in automatic mesh generation. Triangular-shaped elements are also easier to fit into geometrically complex structures. Through the combination of different element orders and topologies, for example parabolic and triangular, could improve the accuracy of a topologically lesser element.

An important ingredient in FEA is the behavior of the individual elements. The predictive accuracy of the model will be influenced by the shapes of the elements used, as any deviation in shape from the "ideal" internal elemental strain function will lead to mathematical inaccuracies. Given that FEA offers an approximation to the exact solution, a numerical result closer to this true value will be achieved if the displacements in a finite element model become increasingly continuous. A few good elements may generate better results than many poorer elements.

7.5. ADVANTAGES AND DISADVANTAGES

The power of the finite element analysis resides principally in its flexibility. The method can be used on a variety of physical problems utilizing commercially available finite element analysis packages. The object investigated can have arbitrary loads, support conditions, and shape. The mesh can be a mixture of elements of various shapes, types, and physical properties. This great adaptability is confined within a single computer program. User-prepared input data controls the selection of problem type, geometry, boundary conditions, element selections, and so on.

Another attractive feature of finite elements is the close physical resemblance between the finite element model and the actual structure (Fig. **31**). The model is not simply an abstraction. This seems especially true in structural mechanics, and may account for finite element analysis having its origins there.

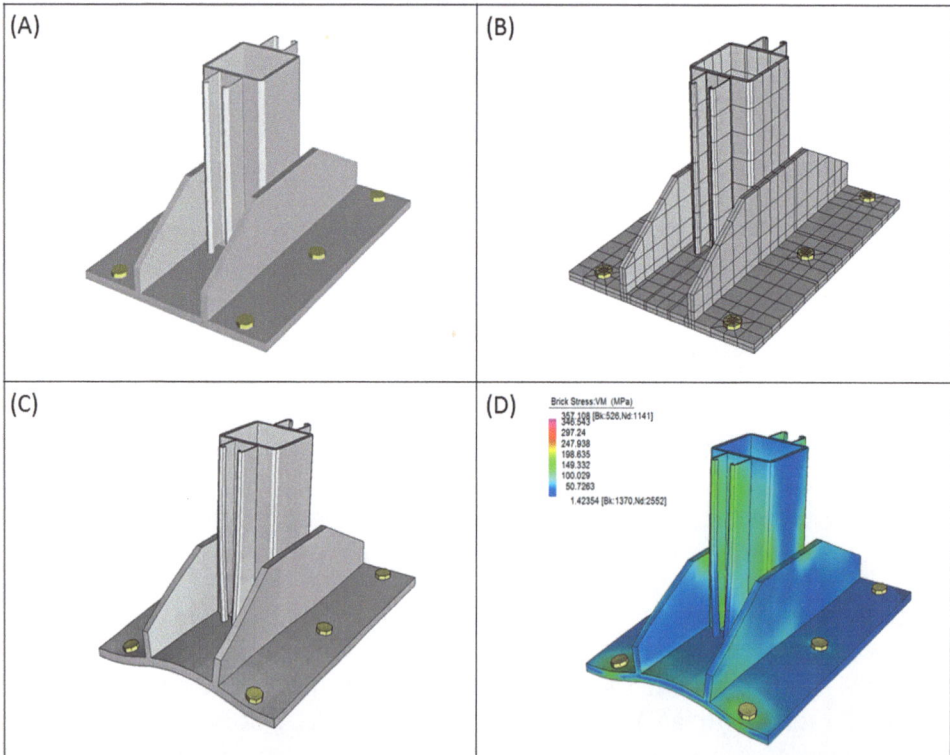

Fig. (31). Solid model (**A**), finite element mesh (**B**), computed deformation (**C**), and von Mises stress (**D**) of a base support.

On the other hand, the finite element approach also has its disadvantages. The finite element approach requires special precaution to be taken during the creation of the wireframe model, because mesh volumes should be generated to provide reasonable geometric aspect ratio and behavior for the derived elements. In theory, a mesh volume could be subdivided into a large number of very small elements to minimize geometric approximation and therefore maximizing model accuracy. On the other hand, this would significantly increase computer processing time and memory requirements. The other possibility is to manipulate the geometry by dividing contoured curves into smaller ones, therefore creating more detailed mesh volumes. Nonetheless, this option is only feasible in regions with anticipated high gradients of material deformation or complex shapes. In doing so, one attempts to build mesh volumes where the creation of a smaller number of elements will provide sufficient accuracy without loss of structural response.

7.6. THE ELEMENT CHARACTERISTIC MATRIX

The element characteristic matrix has different names in different problem areas. In structural mechanics, it is called a stiffness matrix and it relates nodal displacements to nodal forces. In heat conduction, it is called a conductivity matrix and it relates nodal temperatures to nodal fluxes.

There are three important ways to derive an element characteristic matrix:

1. The direct method is based on physical reasoning. It is limited to very simple elements.
2. The variational method is applicable to problems that can be stated by certain integral expressions, such as the expression for potential energy.
3. Weighted residual methods are particularly suited to problems for which differential equations are known but no variational statement is available. For stress analysis and some other problem areas, the variational method and the weighted residual method (the Galerkin method [141, 142]) yield identical finite element formulation.

7.7. MATERIAL PROPERTIES

The assignment of proper material properties to a finite element model is an essential step to guarantee predictive accuracy. Stress and strain within a structure are calculated using the assigned material properties. These properties can be categorized as isotropic, transversely isotropic, orthotropic, and anisotropic.

For an isotropic material, the properties are the same in all directions and since the elastic modulus, the shear modulus, and the Poisson's ratio are interrelated, only two out of the three variables need to be determined for the elastic behavior to be completely characterized. A material is anisotropic if its properties are different when evaluated in different directions. Transversely isotropic materials behave in the same way in every direction about a single axis of symmetry.

An orthotropic material is an anisotropic material that exhibits extreme values of stiffness in mutually perpendicular directions. These directions are called principal directions of the material. An example is wood cut from a log, which is least stiff in the circumferential direction, stiffest in the axial direction, and of intermediate stiffness in the radial direction. If x, y, and z are principal directions, then normal stresses σ_x, σ_y, and σ_z are independent of shear strains γ_{xy}, γ_{yz}, γ_{zx}. The elastic modulus for an orthotropic material contains only nine independent co-efficients. In contrast, a material is anisotropic if its properties are different when measured in different directions.

7.8. NON-LINEAR ANALYSIS

A problem is non-linear if the force-displacement relationship is dependent on the current state of the displacement, force, and stress-strain relations [143]. The force-displacement relation for a non-linear problem can be written as:

$$\{F\} = [K(F, d)]\{d\} \tag{20}$$

where *[K]* is the stiffness matrix, *{F}* is the generalized force vector, and *{d}* is the generalized displacement vector.

Non-linearity in structures can be classed as:

1. Material non-linearity;
2. Geometric non-linearity; and
3. Non-linearity induced by boundary conditions.

In heat transfer, non-linearity may arise from temperature-dependent conductivity and from radiation.

A material is referred to as non-linear if stresses $\{\sigma\}$ and strains $\{\varepsilon\}$ are connected by a strain-dependent matrix rather than a matrix of constants. Consequently, the computational difficulty is that equilibrium equations must be written using material properties that depend on strains, but strains are not known in advance. Plastic flow is often a cause of material non-linearity.

Geometric non-linearity occurs if the relationships of forces and stresses are non-linear with displacements and strains. This can result in loss of structural stability and changes in structural behavior. Examples include large displacement and buckling problems.

Boundary conditions can result in non-linearity if they vary with displacement of the structure. This condition exists when the load and the resistance to the deformation induced by the loads that represent the effects of the surrounding environment on the model. Many of these non-linear boundary conditions have a discontinuous character, which makes them some of the most severe non-linearities in mechanics. Examples are contact and frictional slip effects.

The main difference between linear and non-linear finite element analyses lies in the solution of the algebraic equations. Non-linear analysis is usually more complex and expensive than linear analysis. Non-linear problems generally require an iterative incremental solution strategy to ensure that equilibrium is satisfied at the end of each step. Results from non-linear analysis are not always unique compared to linear problems.

The classifications "linear" and "non-linear" are artificial in that physical reality presents various problems, some of which can be satisfactorily approximated by linear equations. It is fortunate that linear approximations are quite good for many problems of stress analysis and heat conduction. Non-linear approximations are more difficult to formulate, and solving the resulting equations may cost ten to hundred times as much as a linear approximation having the same number of degrees of freedom.

Many physical situations present non-linearities too large to be ignored. Stress-strain relations may be non-linear in either a time-dependent or a time-independent way. A change in configuration may cause loads to alter their distribution and magnitude or cause gaps to open or close. Mating parts may stick or slip. Welding and casting processes cause the material to change in conductivity, modulus, and phase. The generation and shedding of vortices in fluid flow past a structure produce oscillatory loads on the structure. Pre-buckling rotations alter the effective stiffness of a shell and change its buckling load. Consequently, we see that non-linear effects may alter in type and can be mild or severe.

A finite element analyst must be familiar with the physical problem and must be acquainted with different solution strategies. A single strategy will not always work well and may not work at all for some problems. Several attempts may be needed in order to obtain a satisfactory result.

7.9. CONVERGENCE TEST

The accuracy of the finite element analysis can only be quantitatively determined using a convergence test. The test measures how well the mathematics has been approximated. In general, the approximate solution improves as a series of meshes gets more and more refined in a procedure commonly referred to as h-convergence. As more nodes and elements are used, the calculated displacement at any particular node approaches the exact (but generally unknown) displacement solution.

CHAPTER 8

Patient Matching

Abstract: The ability to extract data from computed tomography (CT) or any other appropriate imaging technology to generate the patient's own model is already a common practice. For example, by integrating computerized modeling with medical imaging, it would be possible to determine the correct location, configuration, size and number of implants needed to address the patient's functional and restorative needs. Furthermore, this approach can be used to define the form and mechanical requirements of implants and prostheses employed in the treatment of mandibular and maxillary fractures with fixation and reduction of the fracture obtained with minimal osteosynthesis plate bulk, number and size. This integrated system can be coupled with modern rapid prototyping such as 3D printing and laser sintering to produce superstructures and patient matched dental devices and guides.

Keywords: Bone density, Cancellous bone, Cortical bone, Computed tomography, CT, Elastic properties, Finite element analysis, Finite element modeling, Hounsfield unit, Material properties, Strength.

From a clinical perspective, the usefulness of FEA as a biomechanical foundation in the construction of a predictive tool is ideal for determining the influence of a specific implant design on the degree of osseointegration and remodeling and avoid any potential problems such as bone resorption and stress shielding according to patients' anatomical conditions such as muscle forces and mandibular bone tissues.

8.1. MODEL DEVELOPMENT

The utilization of this computerized modeling methodology will have innumerable applications in both dentistry and in oral and maxillofacial surgery, at not only a research level but also at a clinical level. For example, the creation of a computer model based on data from computed tomography (CT) scans and micro-computed tomography (μ-CT) or other appropriate imaging technique such as, magnetic resonance imaging (MRI) of individual patient is becoming a common practice. This is achieved through the importation of the image data into specialized modeling software where this information is converted into two-dimensional or three-dimensional finite element meshes (Fig. **32**).

Andy H. Choi and Besim Ben-Nissan
All rights reserved-© 2018 Bentham Science Publishers

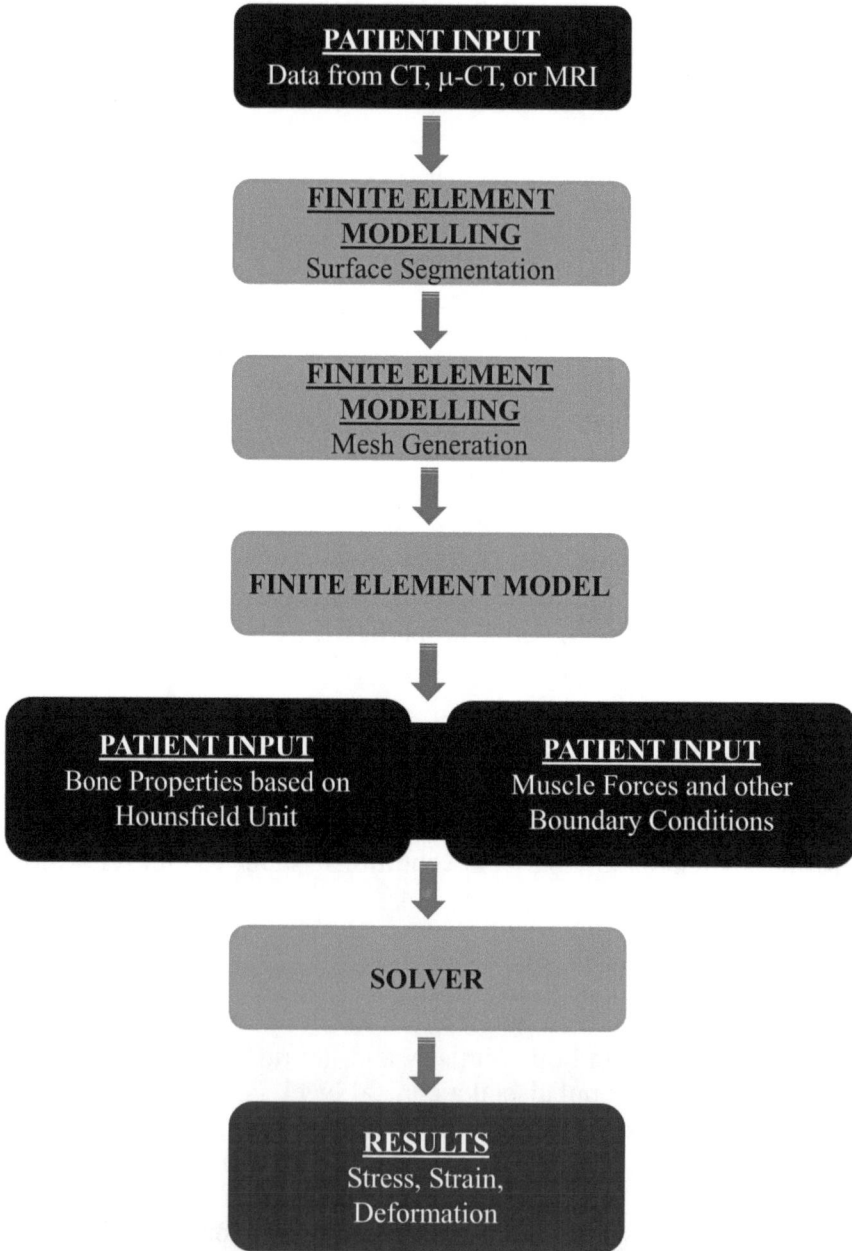

Fig. (32). Schematic showing the process used in the construction and analysis of a patient-specific finite element model.

8.2. MATERIAL PROPERTIES

As discussed in a previous section, the proper assignment of bone material properties is vital as it will greatly affect the distributions of stresses and deformations within a structure. A suitable approximation of the distribution of bone material can be acquired through the use of computed tomography scans. This approach ensures in a more relevant physiological model on a subject specific basis.

According to a study by Rho *et al.* [144], the raw CT values can be converted into Hounsfield Units (H) by relating the bone values to water where the value of H is 0 and to air where the value of H is -1000 [145] using the following equation:

$$H = 1000\frac{CT - CT_{water}}{CT_{water} - CT_{air}} \tag{21}$$

Bone density is defined as mean value expressed in Hounsfield units in each pixel.

The apparent density of bone ($\rho_{apparent}$) can be calculated using a linear equation from Hounsfield units [146, 147]:

$$\rho_{apparent} = a + bH \tag{22}$$

The values of *a* and *b* are determined using a linear calibration derived from two reference points in one of the CT scan slices. The first reference point should represent non-bone condition in which the density should be equal to 0 g/cm^3. The second reference point can be of cortical or compact bone with an averaged density of 1.768 g/cm^3 according to a study by Dechow *et al.* [57] recorded from 17 mandible samples or 1.85 to 2.0 g/cm^3 according to studies by Schwartz-Dabney and Dechow [59, 148] from both edentulous and dentate human mandibular cortical bones. The CT gray values from both of the reference points are then substituted into eq. (22) along with the apparent density values. Once the values of *a* and *b* are determined, the apparent density can be calculated at any point in bone using linear interpolation of the raw CT gray values.

Since the late 1970s, extensive investigations have been carried out to examine the relationship between apparent density and the elastic modulus of human cortical and cancellous bone and these mathematical relationships are considerably different from each other [149]. Studies by Carter and co-workers [150, 151] suggested a power-law relationship could be used to determine the elastic modulus (*E*) of both cortical and cancellous bone based on the apparent density:

$$E = A\rho_{apparent}^{B} \tag{23}$$

where A and B are constants derived experimentally. According, eq. (23) can be rearranged to give:

$$\log E = \log A + B \log \rho_{apparent} \tag{24}$$

Therefore, a linear relationship exists between elastic modulus and density when $\log E$ is plotted against $\log \rho$ on a graph. The value of B is the gradient or the slop of the line, while $\log A$ is the intercept with the y-axis. They concluded that the axial elastic modulus (in GPa) is determined by the apparent density to the third power and the strain rate ($\dot{\varepsilon}$) to the power of 0.06. Hence, eq. (23) can be rewritten as:

$$E = 3.79\dot{\varepsilon}^{0.06}\rho_{apparent}^{3} \tag{25}$$

where the apparent density is in g/cm³ and $\dot{\varepsilon}$ is in inverse seconds. They concluded that the power-law relationship is shown to be valid for all bones within the skeleton. This also allows for meaningful predictions of strength and stiffness of bone tissues based on *in vivo* density measurements.

Later, a statistical analysis of the pooled data from a number of previous experiments concerning the dependence of the elastic modulus of cancellous bone tissue and apparent density was presented by Rice *et al.* [152]. Their findings revealed that the elastic modulus is proportional to the square of apparent density of the tissue.

- In the longitudinal direction:

$$E_{compression} = 0.06 + 0.90\rho_{apparent}^{2} \tag{26}$$

$$E_{tension} = 0.06 + 1.65\rho_{apparent}^{2} \tag{27}$$

- In the transverse direction:

$$E_{compression} = 0.06 - 0.15\rho_{apparent}^{2} \tag{28}$$

$$E_{tension} = 0.06 + 0.60\rho_{apparent}^{2} \tag{29}$$

A study by Schaffler and Burr revealed that the stiffness of compact bone was found to be highly and nonlinearly dependent on its porosity, its complement, bone volume fraction and apparent density [153]. Elastic modulus decreases as a power of increasing porosity and increases both as a power of increasing bone tissue volume and increasing apparent density. The relationship between elastic modulus (E) in GPa and apparent density (ρ) in g/cm^3 is:

$$E = 0.09\rho_{apparent}^{7.4}$$ (30)

In the mid-1990s, Rho *et al.* [144] examined the possibility of developing bone specific relationships that can be used to predict the elastic modulus from CT numbers and density in human bone. Seventy-two samples of cortical bones from the mandible were obtained: three transverse sections at 40%, 60% and 80% of the total bone length and three annular specimens originated from the buccal, lingual and inferior aspects of the mandibular corpus. The increasing percentage in bone length represents positions from the chin to the ramus. Based on their findings, three linear relations for cortical bone between elastic modulus expressed in GPa and density (ρ) expressed in kg/m^3 were derived:

$$E_{radial} = 6.382 + 0.255\, E_{superior-inferior}$$ (31)

$$E_{radial} = -13.05 + 0.013\, \rho$$ (32)

$$E_{superior-inferior} = -23.93 + 0.024\, \rho$$ (33)

Hodgskinson and Currey proposed a regression that can be used to describe the relationship between the elastic modulus (in MPa) and the apparent density (in kg/m^3) of human cancellous bone [154]:

$$Mean\ E = 0.004\rho_{apparent}^{1.96}$$ (34)

A study by Keller proposed the elastic modulus (GPa) of both cortical and cancellous bone could be calculated using the ash density (g/cm^3), which is determined by dividing the bone ash mass by the total specimen volume, using the following power-law relationship [155]:

$$E = 10.5\rho_{ash}^{2.57}$$ (35)

Using specimens of human trabecular bones from various anatomic sites, power-law regressions between elastic modulus (GPa) and apparent density (g/cm^3) were derived by Morgan *et al.* [156]:

$$E = 7.540\rho_{apparent}^{1.72} \tag{36}$$

The reported range:

$$E = 10.55\rho_{apparent}^{1.94} \tag{37}$$

The mean regression reported when the data from all anatomic sites were pooled:

$$E = 8.920\rho_{apparent}^{1.83} \tag{38}$$

Table 10. Summary of the relationships between the elastic modulus and density as described in the text.

Investigators		E	ρ
All Bone Types			
Carter *et al.*	$E = 3.79\dot{\varepsilon}^{0.06}\rho_{apparent}^3$	GPa	g/cm^3
Keller	$E = 10.5\rho_{ash}^{2.57}$	GPa	g/cm^3
Cortical Bone			
Schaffler & Burr	$E = 0.09\rho_{apparent}^{7.4}$	GPa	g/cm^3
Rho *et al.*	$E_{radial} = 6.382 + 0.255\,E_{superior-inferior}$ $E_{radial} = -13.05 + 0.013\,\rho$ $E_{superior-inferior} = -23.93 + 0.024\,\rho$	GPa	kg/m^3
Cancellous Bone			
Rice	Longitudinal Direction $E_{compression} = 0.06 + 0.90\rho_{apparent}^2$ $E_{tension} = 0.06 + 1.65\rho_{apparent}^2$ Transverse Direction $E_{compression} = 0.06 - 0.15\rho_{apparent}^2$ $E_{tension} = 0.06 + 0.60\rho_{apparent}^2$		
Hodgskinson & Currey	$Mean\ E = 0.004\rho_{apparent}^{1.96}$	MPa	kg/m^3
Morgan *et al.*	$E = 7.540\rho_{apparent}^{1.72}$ $E = 8.920\rho_{apparent}^{1.83}$ $E = 10.55\rho_{apparent}^{1.94}$	GPa	g/cm^3

As mentioned in a review by Poelert *et al.* [157], the biggest challenge is determining which power law regression is the most accurate (Table **10**). Furthermore, a study has revealed that a slightly more accurate result can be obtained when one single value of density, and therefore elastic modulus, is assigned to every element (conventional technique) than compared to changing the values of density and mechanical properties within the same element (modified technique) [158].

8.3. MUSCLE FORCES AND OTHER BOUNDARY CONDITIONS

Given the fact that muscular forces cannot be measured directly under non-invasive conditions, it is vital to determine the appropriate magnitude of the muscle forces used in a patient-specific mathematical model for studying the *in vivo* biomechanical behavior of bones, and in particular the mandible (Fig. **33**) [159].

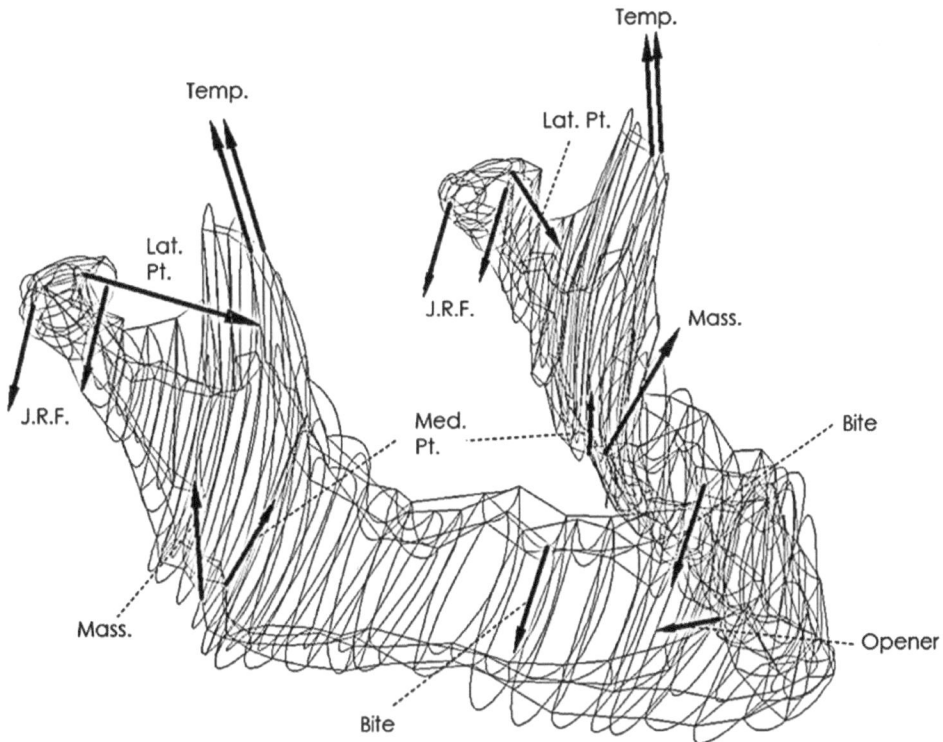

Fig. (33). Applied forces during simulated clenching [160]. (Bite) Bite force; (Mass.) Masseter; (Med. Pt.) Medial Pterygoid; (Temp.) Temporalis; (Lat. Pt.) Lateral Pterygoid; (J.R.F.) Joint Reaction Force.

The following steps are used to estimate the force magnitudes of masticatory muscles during various functional movements of the mandible such as clenching, opening, and protrusion [160, 161]:

1. All the forces are assumed to be symmetrical with respect to the mid-line and to have an equal magnitude on the right and left side of the mandible.
2. The forces exerted by contracting muscles are represented by vectors. The direction of these vectors can be defined by the connecting lines between the centroids of the origins and the insertions of the muscles.
3. The value of maximum muscle tension, which directly relates to its physiological cross-sectional area, is used to determine the maximum force that a muscle can exert.
4. The lines of masticatory muscle actions and their moment arms are determined.
5. The moments generated by the sum of the applied muscle and bite forces must be equal to the moment generated by the reaction forces applied at the condylar region.

8.4. APPLICATIONS

This model can then be used in the following applications:

1. **Dental Implants**: It is possible to determine the correct number, location, size and configuration of implants needed to address that person's functional and restorative needs. In such instance, the dentist or dental clinician is able to predict the functional loads that an implant-supported cantilevered bridge restoration may develop based on the patient's own muscle forces and bone properties. Consequently, the clinician can plan any necessary implant surgery in an attempt to predictably provide support for the potential loads. In doing so, the chance of failure can be minimized, and likewise, the potential of over-treatment. Furthermore, through the use of mathematical algorithms, it is possible to describe bone formation and remodeling induced by dental implants.
2. **Restorative Dentistry:** In a similar context to dental implant restorations, various restorative tooth options can be examined under simulated functional loading and designed to resist these loads prior to manufacturing.
3. **Temporomandibular Joint Surgery**: In the past, intense scrutiny has been placed on temporomandibular joint prostheses as a result of breakdowns caused mainly by material failure. It is expected that patient requiring temporomandibular joint replacement can benefit from improvements in the design and material used in these prostheses based on computational simulations. In addition, computational modeling technology can also

contribute to *in vitro* testing of these prostheses by refining its design so that damages caused by a number of materials failures in the past can be avoided.

4. **Distraction Osteogenesis:** The success of distraction osteogenesis of the mandible is dependent on the accurate planning of the distraction vector needed to produce the final position of the distracted segment. At present, patient-matched computational modeling can be combined with finite element analysis to refine this planning process, and in particular, as the use of intraoral multi-directional distraction devices becomes widespread.

5. **Aesthetic Facial Surgery:** In addition to refining the process of surgical planning, patient-matched computational modeling can also be applied to examine different aspects of facial bone osteotomies such as post-operative functional change and stability of the orthognathic movements.

6. **Pathology Resection and Reconstruction:** Reconstructions after the resection of various pathologies involving the mandible can be carried out using patient-matched modeling so that function and form are returned to the premorbid state as closely as possible.

7. **Traumatology:** Accurate patient-matched three-dimensional modeling will allow surgeons and clinicians to best determine the form and engineering requirements of hardware such as plates that is utilized in the treatment of injuries such as mandibular fractures. This means that both reduction and fixation of the fracture can be achieved while at the same time minimizing the number and size of the osteosynthesis plates used. More importantly, patient-matched modeling in conjunction with mathematical modeling such as finite element analysis has been used to simulate the bone remodeling and healing process of bone fractures. Computational models of the fracture healing process may prove useful in the determination of optimal mechanical-based treatments after an accident, trauma, or a fall.

CHAPTER 9

Bone Fracture Healing

Abstract: The bone remodeling sequence is composed of three consecutive phases: resorption, reversal, and formation. The utilization of numerical models to simulate the fracture healing process may prove to be advantageous in determining the ideal mechanical-based reconstruction or treatment after an illness or accident.

Keywords: Bone remodeling, Finite element analysis, FEA, Osteoclasts, Osteoblasts.

It has been accepted that the principle behind the bone remodeling sequence is to sustain the integrity of the skeleton. This is achieved through the collaborative efforts of osteoclasts and osteoblasts, the constituent cells of bone. The origin of osteoblast cells can be traced back to multipotent mesenchymal stem cells (MSCs), which possess the ability to separate into osteoblasts as well as into adipocytes, chondrocytes, fibroblasts and myoblasts [162, 163]. The osteoblasts are responsible for the production of bone matrix constituents and are discovered in clusters along the bone surface, "coating" the layer of bone matrix they are creating [163]. On the other hand, the osteoclasts are responsible for bone resorption. They are derived from hematopoietic cells of the mononuclear lineage and are giant multinucleated cells with a diameter of up to 100 nm [164].

9.1. BONE REMODELING PROCESS

The close collaboration between osteoblasts and osteoclasts in the remodeling process is often termed basic multicellular unit. Bone resorption and bone formation are balanced in a homeostatic equilibrium. On a cellular level, the simultaneous mechanical and biological actions play a governing role in the delicate equilibrium between bone growth, formation and resorption. In addition, the combination of the osteoblasts and osteoclasts also contributes to the bone remodeling of defects such as micro-fractures [165].

The bone remodeling sequence is composed of three consecutive phases: resorption, reversal and formation. The resorption phase initiates with the migra-tion of partially differentiated mononuclear pre-osteoclasts to the bone surface for

Andy H. Choi and Besim Ben-Nissan

the formation of multinucleated osteoclasts. The appearance of mononuclear cells on the bone surface as well as the commencement of osteoclastic resorption marks the beginning of the reversal phase. Mononuclear cells provide signals for the differentiation and migration of osteoblasts and create surfaces for new osteoblasts to begin bone formation. The final phase is the formation phase and it occurs when the resorbed bone is replaced completely with the new bone deposited by osteoblasts. Flattened lining cells cover the entire surface once the formation phase is completed. A prolonged resting period will take place until the beginning of a new remodeling sequence [163].

The utilization of numerical models to simulate the fracture healing process may prove to be advantageous in determining the ideal mechanical-based reconstruction or treatment after an illness or accident. Through the combined use of a mechanoregulation algorithm and a discrete lattice modeling, the cellular processes involved in healing such as the apoptosis, differentiation, migration and proliferation of cells were studied by Byrne *et al.* [166] in an attempt to simulate bone regeneration under realistic muscle loading.

9.2. CURRENT DEVELOPMENT

A number of investigators reported mathematical modeling by the finite element simulation which predicted the key phases of fracture healing [166 - 168]. Furthermore, by incorporating the transition of woven bone into lamellar bone, the authors simulated bone healing beyond the reparative phase. In a relative study by Grivas *et al.* [168], the limitations of FEA in the prediction of cell proliferation during bone healing were addresses. Numerical simulations of cell diffusions were derived in a 2-D model using a new meshless local boundary integral equation approach.

Experimental studies have revealed that one of the primary mechanisms for the course of bone healing is interfragmentary movement despite the fact that there are also other factors that will have an effect on fracture healing [169].

The effectiveness of computational models to resolve the complex relations between tissue formation and mechanical environment was first suggested by García-Aznar *et al.* [170] and later in a study by Comiskey *et al.* [171] where they analyzed callus formation for two cases of bone fracture healing. Compressive strain field experienced by the immature callus tissue as a result of interfragmentary movement was determined using plane strain models of the oblique fractures. The external formation of calluses was derived using an optimization algorithm which iteratively eliminates tissue that experiences low strains from a large domain. Recently, a combined failure-repair mechanistic computation model was suggested by Alierta *et al.* [169] to describe the healing process of a bone fracture. The bone fracture gap was generated in the model using interface elements to connect the two fracture ends and to simulate the discontinuity in the displacement field between fragments.

Although the works mentioned above are centered on numerical simulations of fracture healing processes in long bones such as the femur, the same principle can be applied to an oral environment. Above all, investigations have been carried out to predict the possibility of bone formation and remodeling as well as the risk of further bone fracture induced by fixation plates used in the treatment of mandibular fractures [172 - 178]. Recently, the conditions for good and rapid bone healing induced by mini-plate for osteosynthesis of mandibular angle fracture were examined in a study by Pituru *et al.* [178]. In their work, they designed a mini-plate that attempts to keep the maximum strains generated in the cortical bone (near the fracture line) during accidental biting to a magnitude below the threshold causing bone resorption while offering maximum fracture stability. The operational effectiveness of the mini-plate was confirmed with a three-dimensional finite element model.

It has been well established that immobilization or the absence of excessive mobility is crucial for the unification of the fracture segments and this stability plays an influential role for the healing of soft and hard tissues in the injured or fractured area. This implies that the fracture site must be stabilized to aid in the physiological process toward normal bony healing using mechanical means [174]. A study by Joshi and Kurakar [174] suggested that bone healing would be problematic if the gap between the fracture fragments is more than 0.15 mm after reduction and fixation, which ultimately leads to failure of treatment. Bone interfragmentary displacement during various loading conditions was examined when the mandible fracture segments were treated with different designs of mini-plates. In another study, various fixation schemes used to fixate mandibular angle fractures were biomechanically evaluated by Kimsal *et al.* [172]. Principal strains in the callus at the fracture site were used to assess the ideal fixation candidate as a less invasive fixation approach to fractures of the mandibular angle.

CHAPTER 10

Bone Remodeling - Dental Implants

Abstract: During functional movements such as chewing, forces on the prosthesis will be transferred to the implants and this will result in stresses being generated within the bone surrounding the implants. The bone-implant interface is of great significance to osseointegration as the utilization of dental implants may alter the mechanical environment of the mandible. Bone remodeling occurs in the first year of function in response to occlusal forces and establishment of the normal dimensions of the peri-implant soft tissues. The type of bone remodeling taking place in the bone tissue surrounding the implant will be governed by the variations in the internal stress state. Stress shielding and bone resorption will occur when no load is being transferred to the supporting tissues, while abnormally high stress concentration can lead to implant failure. For these reasons, it is essential to consider the effect of bone remodeling on the performance of dental implants and prostheses in order to improve its efficiency. The bone remodeling process around dental implants has been simulated in a number of studies using a variety of models. Mathematical algorithms such as nano-interactions and mechanosensory mechanisms have been incorporated into numerical models to describe bone formation and osseointegration of dental implants. Furthermore, strain energy density algorithm has been adapted to illustrate bone remodeling induced by implants and fixed partial dentures.

Keywords: Adaptive bone remodeling, Bone-implant interface, Bone remodeling, Lazy zone, Stanford theory, Strain energy density SED, Stress shielding.

During mandibular movement, the interface between implant and bone is of great significance to osseointegration as the utilization of dental implants may alter the mechanical environment of the mandible. This may also lead to the remodeling and adaptation of the surrounding cortical and cancellous bone tissues. Consequently, it is vital that the influence of bone remodeling on the longevity of implants and devices be considered in an effort to enhance its efficacy [179].

During functional movements such as chewing, forces on the prosthesis will be transferred to the implants and this will result in stresses being generated within the bone surrounding the implants. Bone remodeling occurs in the first year of function in response to occlusal forces and establishment of the normal dimensions of the peri-implant soft tissues. The type of bone remodeling, *i.e.*

Andy H. Choi and Besim Ben-Nissan

constructive or destructive, taking place in the bone tissue surrounding the implant will be governed by the variations in the internal stress state.

Stress shielding and bone resorption will occur when no load is being transferred to the supporting tissues, while abnormally high stress concentration can lead to implant failure. For these reasons, it is essential to consider the effect of bone remodeling on the performance of dental implants and prostheses in order to improve its efficiency.

A number of factors are involved in the achievement of osseointegration and these include material composition, design and geometry of implant, adequate bone quality and interface interactions, and absence of overheating during site preparation and surgical technique.

The bone remodeling process around dental implants has been simulated in a number of studies using a variety of models (Fig. **34**). Mathematical algorithms such as nano-interactions and mechanosensory mechanisms have been incorporated into numerical models to describe bone formation and osseointegration of dental implants. Furthermore, strain energy density algorithm has been adapted to illustrate bone remodeling induced by implants and fixed partial dentures.

10.1. STRAIN ENERGY DENSITY

The development of mathematical theory for bone remodeling was first initiated in the 1970's with the theory of adaptive elasticity [180, 181]. Afterward, an investigation was carried out using a similar theory on the relationship between long-term adaptive bone remodeling and orthopedic implants in both 2-D and 3-D finite element models [180]. The shape or bone density adaptations to various functional requirements were regulated by the strain energy density as a feedback control variable.

In their study, strain energy density (SED) was expressed in the general form of:

$$SED = \frac{1}{2}\, \varepsilon_{ij}\!:\sigma_{ij} \tag{39}$$

Where, ε_{ij} and σ_{ij} are the components of the local strain and stress tensors and when it was applied to bone remodeling, the strain energy density describes the rate of variation in bone density (ρ) using the relation:

$$\frac{\partial \rho}{\partial t} = C\,(SED_{actual} - SED_{homeostatic}) \tag{40}$$

The homeostatic SED ($SED_{homeostatic}$) is referred to as the local actual strain energy density and the driving force for adaptive activity was postulated to be the difference between the actual strain energy density (SED_{actual}) and a site-specific homeostatic equilibrium SED ($SED_{homeostatic}$), and C quantifies the rate of adaptation. A "lazy zone" as previously suggested by Carter [182] assumed that a certain threshold level in over- or under-loading must be exceeded before bone reacts.

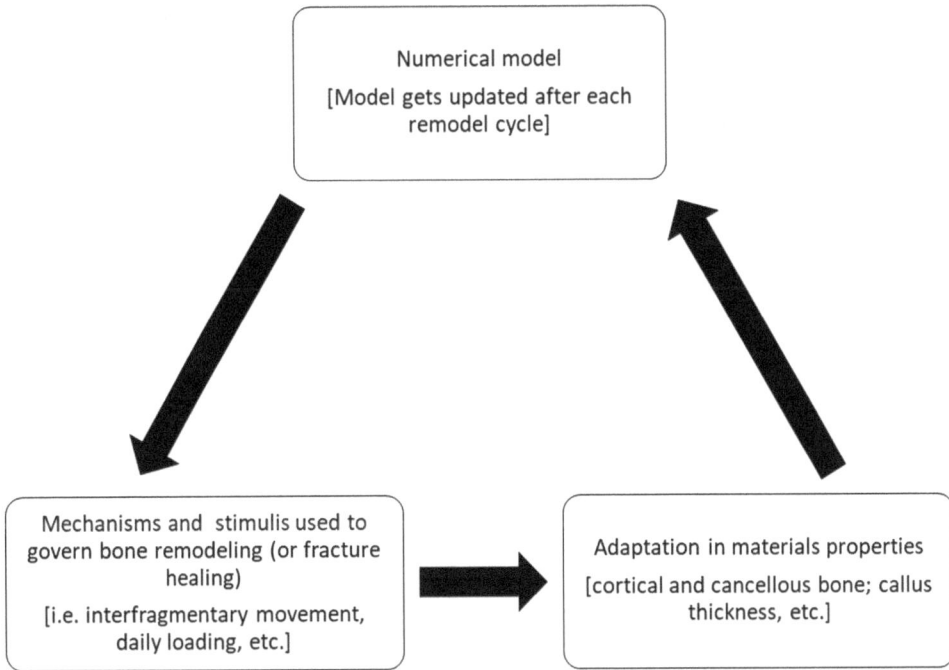

Fig. (34). Basic schematic representations of the steps involved in bone remodeling calculation using FEA. Modified from [167].

Adaptive activity is initiated if:

$$SED_{actual} > (1+s)SED_{homeostatic} \qquad (41)$$

or

$$SED_{actual} < (1-s)SED_{homeostatic} \qquad (42)$$

where s is the threshold level, and the rate of variation in bone density in the "lazy zone" which can be defined as:

$$\frac{\partial \rho}{\partial t} = \begin{cases} C[SED_{actual} - SED_{homeostatic}(1+s)] \\ 0 \\ C[SED_{actual} - SED_{homeostatic}(1-s)] \end{cases} \tag{43}$$

if

$$\begin{aligned} SED_{actual} &> SED_{homeostatic}(1+s) \\ (1-s)SED_{homeostatic} \leq SED_{actual} &\leq (1+s)SED_{homeostatic} \\ SED_{actual} &< SED_{homeostatic}(1-s) \end{aligned}$$

The same strain energy density algorithm was used in a number of bone remodeling studies induced by dental implants and was selected as the mechanical stimulus initially in 2004 by Mellal *et al.* to investigate the stresses at the implant-bone interface before and after osseointegration [183]. It was, then used to examine the preliminary bone remodeling around implants placed in the maxilla [184] and in a post-extraction socket [185] under different loading conditions. It was also used in a hypothetical study where the relationship between low-stiffness implants and stress shielding was examined [186]. Marginal bone loss around low-stiffness implants were determined by applying the calculated strain energy density values to the "lazy zone" range as suggested by Huiskes *et al.* [180].

In addition, studies have also been carried out on fixed partial dentures (FPD) to examine the relationship between biomechanics and bone remodeling caused by different abutments and configurations [187, 188]. It was also hypothesized in a recent study that the combination of medical imaging such as positron emission tomography (PET) and FEA containing mechanobiological stimuli such as strain energy density could present a new approach to clinically monitor and examine bone remodeling driven by fixed partial dentures [189].

10.2. STANFORD THEORY

Originally developed by Carter [190] and further extended by Beaupré and co-workers [191], the so-called "Stanford theory" is a time-dependent approach for emulating bone modeling and remodeling in response to the daily loading history.

In their work, the daily tissue level stress stimulus (ψ_b) was defined by the following equation:

$$\psi_b = \left(\sum_d n_i \sigma_i^m \right)^{\frac{1}{m}} \tag{44}$$

where n_i is the number of cycles of load type i, and m is the stress component.

The continuum level effective stress (σ_i) can be defined as:

$$\sigma_i = \sqrt{2EU} \tag{45}$$

where U is the continuum strain energy density and E is the continuum average elastic modulus. Furthermore, they devised an equation applicable to both external and internal remodeling, which can be used directly to determine the bone apposition or resorption rate on external surfaces. The bone apposition or resorption rate ($\dot{r}$) can be expressed as:

$$\left(\frac{\mu m}{day}\right) = \begin{cases} (\psi_b - \psi_{b.as})c + c \cdot w \\ 0 \\ (\psi_b - \psi_{b.as})c - c \cdot w \end{cases} \tag{46}$$

$$\text{if}$$

$$\begin{array}{c} [(\psi_b - \psi_{b.as}) < -w] \\ [-w \leq (\psi_b - \psi_{b.as})] \leq w \\ [(\psi_b - \psi_{b.as}) > w] \end{array}$$

where c is the empirical rate constant, w is half the width of the central, normal activity region, and $\psi_{b.as}$ is the average daily tissue level attractor state stimulus.

This algorithm was then adopted to predict the time-dependent bone remodeling around dental implants with various macro-geometric designs and lengths [192, 193] and in reduced bone width [194].

10.3. ADAPTIVE BONE REMODELING

It has been previously described that the mechanobiological sensors within the bone can detect mechanical stimuli. The bone will respond by adapting its morphology once there is a deviation in the mechanical loading from the specific homeostatic level [195, 196].

A study by Wang *et al.* [197] combined adaptive bone remodeling with microdamage-based mechanosensory mechanisms to examine the remodeling behavior of trabecular architecture around dental implants. Their study was based on the value of damage accumulation (ω) determined using Miner's rule as suggested by McNamara and Prendergast [198]:

$$\dot{\omega} = \frac{1}{N_f} \tag{47}$$

where N_f is defined as the number of cycles to failure of the material at a given stress level.

According to a study by Carter *et al.* [199], an empirical equation can be used to calculate the value of N_f for bone:

$$\log N_f = H \, \log \sigma^i + J \cdot T + K \cdot \rho^i + M \tag{48}$$

where σ is the stress (MPa), ρ is the density in g/cm^3, and T in °C of the material. H, J, K, and M are empirical constants.

The damage accumulates can then be calculated using:

$$\omega = \int_0^t \dot{\omega}dt \tag{49}$$

where ω is the state of local damage bone tissue, and t is the duration of the calculation.

Strain-adaptive remodeling was considered to be the governing mechanism in the remodeling process when the damage accumulation (ω) is below the critical damage threshold. On the other hand, if the damage accumulation value exceeds the damage threshold, then damage-induced remodeling will take over. The local bone density is changed by the combined algorithms of adaptive and microdamage remodeling. The value of elastic modulus is updated based on the change in the bone density value using an equation derived by Currey [40]:

$$E_i = C\rho_i^n \tag{50}$$

This process is carried out repeatedly to predict the evolution of microarchitecture around four implant systems.

A similar approach was used in the examination of peri-implant bone remodeling and the influence of biomechanical factors such as the properties of osteogenic bone grafts and the magnitude of occlusal loads [200]. In their study, the remodeling process occurs due to biomechanical adjustments imposed by dental implantations and the process continues until the difference between altered state and the homeostatic state, which was based on a model consisted of a natural tooth, is minimized.

10.4. BONE-IMPLANT NANOINTERACTION

Mathematical models using nanointeractions to describe the osseointegration of dental implants and bone formation was first suggested by Moreo *et al*. [201] and later by Vanegas-Acosta *et al*. [202]. Moreo *et al*. proposed a mathematical framework based on a set of reaction-diffusion equations that attempts to model the main biological interactions taking place at the surface of implants. Later, they investigated the influence of variables such as geometry of the implant, cell stimulation, and the initial cell concentration in the host bone on peri-implant bone ingrowth [201].

Vanegas-Acosta *et al*. attempted to formulate a mathematical model via a mechanobiological approach to describe the osseointegration process at the implant-bone interface. In their study, an injury area with a thickness of 1 μm measured from the implant surface was defined for equations related to the concentration of osteogenesis and osteogenic chemical compound that corresponds to the contact zone between the implant surface and the tissues in formation. Their study also assumed that new osteoid formation in the injury area depends on fibrin matrix displacement, and for that reason, the mechanical properties of tissue are related to surface roughness [202].

CHAPTER 11

Dental Bioceramics

Abstract: Bioceramics prior to the 1970s were utilized as implants to perform singular and biologically inert roles. The limitations with these manufactured materials as tissue substitutes were emphasized with the growing realization that tissues and cells of the human body function other different metabolic and regulatory roles. The demands of bioceramics have changed from sustaining a fundamentally physical function without provoking a host response to providing a more positive interaction with the host ever since. This has been complemented by increasing demands on medical devices to extend the duration of life in addition to improving its quality. More importantly, the exciting and potential opportunities associated with the use of nanobioceramics as body interactive materials, facilitating the body to heal, or promoting the regeneration of tissues, therefore restoring physiological functions. Major factors in determining the potential applications of a biomaterial are its biocompatibility and functionality. Furthermore, the bioceramic should not suffer any deformation when loaded under physiological situations. In terms of mechanical properties, the safety of ceramic components is related to their mechanical strength. As a result, improving the mechanical strength of ceramics is the primary objective as well as all the properties which are interrelated to strength.

Keywords: Alumina Al_2O_3, Bioactive glass, Bioceramics, Bioglass, Calcium phosphate, Fracture toughness, Glass ceramics, Hot isostatic pressing, Hot pressing, Hydroxyapatite HAp, Nanobioceramics, Nanocomposites, Partially stabilized zirconia PSZ, Sol-gel, Zirconia ZrO_2, 3-D printing.

The high toughness of metals can generally be derived from their crack-tip plasticity. The fracture energy is absorbed in the plastic zone, creating a tortuous pathway which makes the propagation of the crack much more difficult. Despite the fact that a certain amount of plasticity can also occur at the tip of a crack in a ceramic material, the energy absorption nonetheless is relatively small, resulting in a low fracture toughness value. The values of fracture toughness (K_{IC}) for most ceramics including alumina are roughly one-fiftieth of those of ductile materials such as titanium and its alloys (Table **11**).

Andy H. Choi and Besim Ben-Nissan

Table 11. Mechanical and physical properties of biomaterials [203 - 206].

	Elastic Modulus (GPa)	Tensile Strength (MPa)	Compressive Strength (MPa)	Fracture Toughness (MPa$\bullet$m$^{1/2}$)	Density (g/cm^3)
Human Tissue					
Cartilage	0.002 - 0.01	5 - 25			
Cancellous Bone	0.2 - 0.5	10 - 20	----	----	----
Cortical Bone	3.8 - 11.7	82 - 114	88 - 164	2 - 12	1.7 - 2.0
Metal					
Ti-6Al-4V	114	900 - 1172	450 - 1850	44 - 66	4.43
Bioceramics					
Bioglass ® 45S5	35	42	500	0.7-1.1	----
HAp (3% porosity)	7 - 13	38 - 48	350 - 450	3.05 - 3.15	----
Zirconia (TZP)	210	800 - 1500	1990	6.4 - 10.9	5.74 - 6.08
Alumina (Al$_2$O$_3$)	420	282 - 551	4400	3 - 5.4	3.98

It is important to mention that toughness is an important mechanical property when examining the durability of a biomedical material. It is defined as the materials' capacity to absorb energy during deformation until the point of fracture, normally measured in terms of fracture toughness [203].

11.1. MEDICAL-GRADE BIOCERAMICS

Introduced in the early 1970s, the application of ceramics in the field of maxillofacial and orthopedic implants has brought about the widespread acknowledgment that the proper utilization of ceramics can answer a number of challenges that exist in surgery.

The primary purpose for creating prerequisites governing medical-grade bioceramics is to categorize materials which are bioinert to a human body for a period of more than ten years. According to a study by Willmann [207], the bioceramic must possess a high resistance against corrosion within the human body environment. This can only be achieved through the use of a high-purity oxide ceramic manufactured using purified raw materials which are free of impurities such as silicate and alkaline oxides.

Major factors in determining the potential applications of a biomaterial are its biocompatibility and functionality. Furthermore, the bioceramic should not suffer any deformation when loaded under physiological situations. In terms of mechanical properties, the safety of ceramic components is related to their mechanical strength. As a result, improving the mechanical strength of ceramics is the primary objective as well as all the properties which are interrelated to strength (Table **11**).

Functionality and biocompatibility are related directly to their nanoscale interactions at the bone/implant interface. Improvements of these interfaces using surface modifications and micro- and nanoscale coatings have been of interest worldwide during the past two decades. Currently, a number of companies have started to introduce these new generation nanoscale-modified implants for soft- and hard-tissue engineering into the market for dental, orthopedic, and maxillofacial surgery.

Numerous applications of ceramics are based upon unique mechanical, physical, and thermal properties. In terms of their usage in dentistry and orthopedics, or in biomedical applications in general, their biocompatibility, strength, density, and wear resistance are of vital importance. Density as a physical property is important. Open porosity is often a crucial measurement and is an important density parameter. The porosity of a substance is determined by the volume of pores present in the material and it can have a strong influence on the properties of a ceramic material. The strength of a ceramic can be reduced by open porosity, which also permits the penetrations of liquids or gases into the ceramic. For that reason, it is often important to identify the nature of the porosity as well as determining the density.

Ceramic biomaterials or bioceramics are a category of ceramics that are used in the biomedical field to repair and reconstruct damaged and deceased tissues of musculo-skeletal systems [208]. Different classes of these materials are known based on their response to biological environment. For instance, alumina (Al_2O_3) and zirconia (ZrO_2) are classified as bioinert and bioglass and glass ceramic are bioactive, while calcium phosphate ceramics are classified as bioactive and bio-resorbable (Fig. **35**).

Even though bioceramics are widely used as implants in orthopedics, maxillofacial surgery and for dental implants, more developments are in progress to extend their applications and achieve improvements in their performance and reliability. The method by which these materials are synthesized or produced will govern their properties and applications as well as their performance within the human body.

11.2. NANOBIOCERAMICS AND NANOCOMPOSITES

Once the size and structure of a particular material falls within the range of 1 to 100 nm, it can be referred to as a "nanostructured material". During the past decade, extensive developments of nanotechnology have occurred in the fields of materials science and engineering as a result of this size. However, when it is valued that these nanostructured materials possess the capacity to be integrated and adapted into biomedical devices, such developments has not come as a surprise. This is conceivable as most biological systems such as protein complexes, viruses and membranes display natural nanostructures.

Nanobioceramics, when used as body interactive material, have the potential to assist the human body to rebuild as well as promoting tissue regenerations, thereby reestablishing physiological functions. This approach is being examined in the development of a new generation of nanobioceramics with a broadened range of medical applications. Porous materials are being utilized as bone grafts at an increasing pace due to the fact that they permit the ingrowth of natural bone, and thus providing a strong bond between the graft and bone.

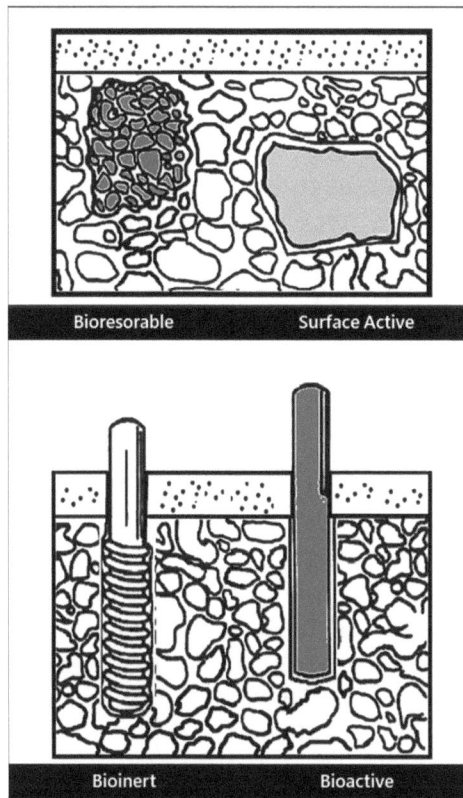

Fig. (35). Classification of bioceramics based on their bioactivity level. Bioresorbable such as tricalcium phosphate implant; surface active such as bioglass or A-W glass; bioinert such as alumina dental implant; bioactive such as hydroxyapatite (HAp) coating on metallic dental implant.

Nanocomposite can be described as a heterogeneous mixture of two or more materials, where at least one of those materials must be on a nanometer-scale. It is possible through the use of the composite approach and the assistance of secondary substitution phases to manipulate the mechanical properties of the composite such as strength and stiffness to a magnitude much closer to the values of natural bone. One such example is hydroxyapatite (HAp)-polymer composite, which has been shown to possess a stiffness value close to that of bone.

Nanocomposites can be synthesized either by physically mixing or through the introduction of a new constituent into an existing nanostructured material. This permits for modifications of the properties of the nanostructured materials and could potentially offer new material functions. The gel system is another form of nanocomposite that has been developed for biomedical applications. In essence, a gel can be thought of as a three-dimensional network immersed in a fluid. Nanostructured materials can be entrapped into a gel such that the properties of the nanomaterials can be enhanced and engineered to match the specific needs of certain biomedical devices.

11.3. CURRENT PRODUCTION TECHNIQUE

The microstructure and properties of ceramic materials including bioceramics and nanoceramics depend in an extreme manner on the production method as well as on their manufacturing route. Subsequently, it is of vital importance to choose the most suitable approach when synthesizing ceramic materials with preferred properties or a combination of properties (Fig. **36**).

The manufacturing approach most widely used for the synthesis of ceramic materials include pressing, in addition to wet chemical processing techniques such as sol-gel and co-precipitation, all of which have been used to produce bioceramics in addition to nanocoatings, nanostructured solid shapes and blocks, and nanoparticles.

In modern ceramics technology, pressing is achieved through the placement of powder into a cast or mold and pressure is applied to reach compaction. Hot pressing and hot isostatic pressing are the most popular techniques used in the manufacture of bioceramics. Hot isostatic pressing can produce higher densities and small grain structures which are essential when it comes to the applications of bioceramics. The process involves the simultaneous applications of heat and pressure. The pressure is applied from all directions *via* a pressurized gas such as argon or helium. In contrast, flat plates or blocks and non-uniform components can be produced with relative ease using hot pressing.

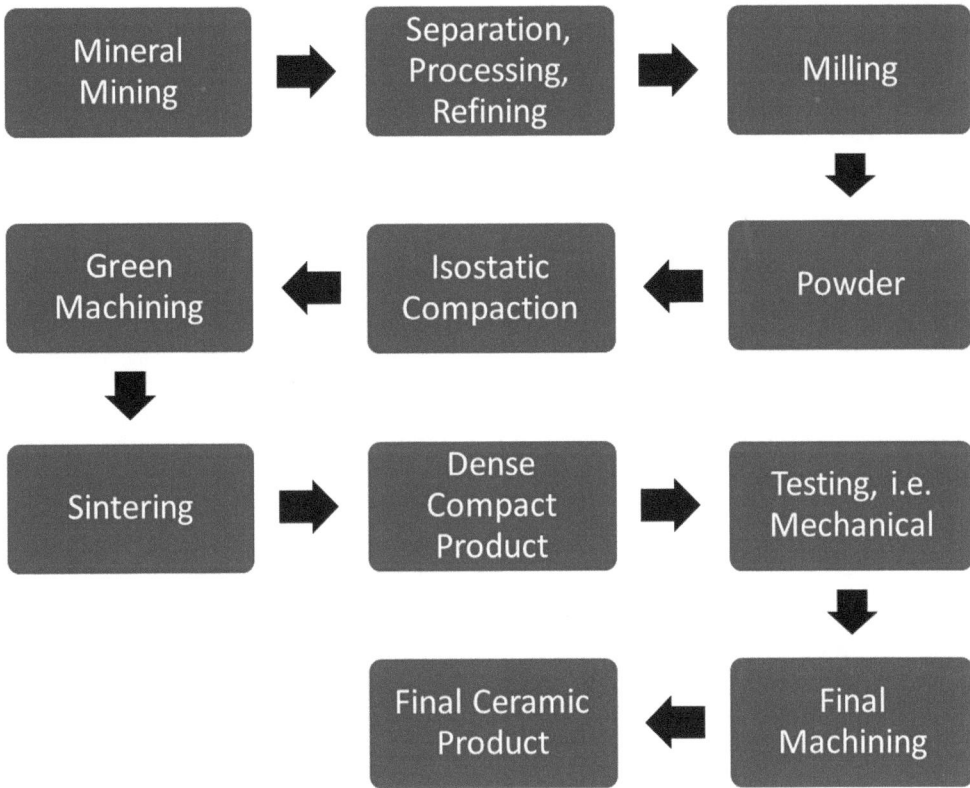

Fig. (36). Schematic showing a typical production process of bioceramics.

11.3.1. Computer-Assisted Design and Manufacturing

Introduced into dentistry in the 1970s and early 1980s, computer-aided designs (CAD) along with computer-assisted manufacturing (CAM) have gained a considerable amount of attention over the past three decades [209 - 211]. Dental restorations and structures can be produced more easily and with greater accuracy using this technology.

In essence, CAD/CAM technology is comprised of three main stages [209 - 212]:

1. Capture of data using imaging technologies such as CT scan. A digitalization tool can also be used to transform geometrical data into digital data to be processed by computer software.
2. Construction of three-dimensional model based on the captured data as well as any other necessary structures such as crowns and abutments using computer design software; and

3. Manufacture of the designed product using a computer-assisted milling and/or grinding unit. Typically, the starting material is a prefabricated block with a range of compositions and materials such as metals (*i.e.* titanium and its alloys), resin materials, and ceramics (*i.e.* alumina and zirconia).

11.3.2. Three-Dimensional (3-D) Printing

Recently, the production of ceramic components with complex shapes is made possible through the introduction of three-dimensional (3D) printing technology. Already established for metals (selective laser melting (SLM)) and polymers (stereolithography, and selective laser sintering (SLS)), 3-D printing has enabled biomedical researchers and engineers to investigate the manufacture of new materials such as bioceramics. Despite the fact that 3-D printing of ceramics is still in its infancy, this technique will be utilized more frequently in the years to come [213].

A number of key advantages are associated with such manufacturing approach including a reduction in the fabrication time as well as in the product costs, and less limitation or constraint placed on the design of the component. Furthermore, an enhancement in dimensional accuracy and surface finish can also be achieved. Similar to CAD/CAM technology, this method can be applied to dentistry as well as oral and maxillofacial surgery and can be used in conjunction with appropriate patient-imaging technology such as CT scans.

In spite of the key advantages, the biggest drawback that needs to be resolved is posed by the materials used. Moreover, partial melting and dissociation of ceramics are serious material issues that need to be thoroughly examined for the 3D printing process. New tools and approaches need to be developed in order to investigate these complex implications. Consequently, improvements in the process and further scientific research are still needed. Furthermore, gaining an in-depth understanding into the interactions between laser and material would enable better control through easier adjustment of the processes' parameters. This in turn will assist in the regulation of residual thermal stress. In most cases, this residual thermal stress causes crack formation and sometimes crumbling of ceramic components produced using 3D printing.

Different to 3D-printed metal and polymer parts, post-treatments are required for ceramic parts created by stereolithography or SLS as they are not "ready-to-use" products. The process typically involves the printed component to undergo thermal treatment to properly remove organic binders used to hold the powders together and sintering at high temperatures that fuses the powders together. This stage is critical if the required physical and mechanical properties are to be achieved in the printed ceramic part.

Without a doubt, post thermal treatments are often needed for components produced stereolithography or SLS and this can lead to dimensional shrinkage that is difficult to predict. In addition, given that the components are constructed layer by layer, the surface of the finished component can suffer from the so-called "staircase effect". This effect can be minimized by building each layer as thin as possible so that it will be difficult to distinguish the various layers. A bad surface finish will require the finished component to undergo grinding or polishing, which add an additional step to the manufacturing procedure. Nevertheless, it is possible to reduce the size of the minimal constitutive element of the printed part and hence the surface finish by optimizing the raw ingredients used, the systems involved in the process, and the process parameters.

11.4. CALCIUM PHOSPHATE

In the search for a suitable biomaterial to substitute and imitate bone, an ideal choice would be synthetic calcium phosphate as they can duplicate the composition and structure of a bone mineral referred to as natural hydroxyapatite. The majority of published data on hydroxyapatite (HAp) is categorized under calcium phosphate to which HAp belongs. As a result, the chemical properties of HAp will be considered from the perspective that it is calcium phosphate despite the fact that it will possess different properties and reactivities from those of other phosphates within the physiological environment.

Calcium phosphate has been widely accepted as a biocompatible material chemically resembling the mineral component of teeth and bone [214 - 216]. Despite the fact of having a similar chemistry as well as composition to that of human bone, the mechanical properties of calcium phosphates are a long way away to those of human bone as a result of their inorganic nature and brittleness. This restricts the use of porous hydroxyapatite in load bearing applications without further modifications.

Calcium phosphates are categorized by specific solubilities, such as when bonded to surrounding tissues along with their capacity to degrade and be replaced by proceeding bone growth. The surface ions of calcium phosphate (or HAp) can be exchanged with those of the aqueous solution when it is exposed to bodily fluid. In contrast, various ions and molecules such as proteins and collagen can be adsorbed onto the surface [216].

The solubilities of different calcium phosphate compounds are given in Table **12** and can be represented as follows [217, 218]:

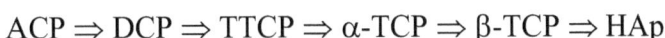

$$ACP \Rightarrow DCP \Rightarrow TTCP \Rightarrow \alpha\text{-TCP} \Rightarrow \beta\text{-TCP} \Rightarrow HAp$$

Calcium phosphate with interconnecting pores in the range of 100 to 500 μm in diameter is commonly used as bone graft materials. The chemistry and structure of calcium phosphate governs its dissolution rates, this in turn determines the *in situ* strength and long-term stability [218 - 220].

In general, it has been acknowledged that synthetic and natural calcium phosphate bioceramics are not osteoinductive, that is, possess the capacity to generate bone once implanted in non-osseous sites, but are osteoconductive, that is, have the ability to support bone formation and tissue ingrowth. The repair of bone and periodontal defects, bone cement additives, ear implants, spine fusion, composites and implant coatings, maxillofacial reconstruction, bone space fillers, alveolar ridge augmentation, artificial eye and ocular implants are just some of the examples where calcium phosphate bioceramics are being utilized in the dental, orthopedic, and medical arenas.

Table 12. Calcium phosphate compounds: abbreviations and chemical formula [218].

Abbreviation	Chemical Compound	Chemical Formula
ACP	Amorphous Calcium Phosphate	
DCP	Dicalcium Phosphate	$CaHPO_4$
TTCP	Tetracalcium Phosphate	$Ca_4O(PO_4)_2$
α-TCP	Tricalcium Phosphate	$Ca_3(PO_4)_2$
β-TCP	Tricalcium Phosphate	$Ca_3(PO_4)_2$
HAp	Calcium Phosphate	$Ca_{10}(PO_4)_6(OH)_2$

Early studies on synthetic apatites and related calcium phosphates were conducted to achieve a better understanding of the composition, properties, and structure of biological apatites, and in particular, human enamel apatites. In spite of this, investigations on synthetic apatites had been centered on their preparation and application in dentistry and medicine as well as their application as scaffolds for teeth and bone regeneration in the past 30 years.

At present, commercially available synthetic calcium phosphate biomaterials are categorized based on their composition. These include α- and β-tricalcium phosphates, HAp, and biphasic calcium phosphate, which is a mixture of β-tricalcium phosphate and HAp with a variable ratio of HAp/β-tricalcium phosphate [218, 220]. Other commercially available calcium phosphate biomaterials have been synthesized from biological materials such as hydrothermally converted coral or derived from marina algae, bovine bone, and processed human bone [216 - 220].

Nanotechnology has created innovative techniques for the manufacture of bone-like synthetic nanocoating and nanopowders of calcium phosphate. The availability of calcium phosphate nanoparticles has indeed created new possibilities in the research and development of high-strength dental and orthopedic nanocomposites and superior biocompatible coatings for implants.

Metal implants like titanium and its alloys have a long-term problem of loosening after being implanted due to a lack of sufficient bioactivity on the surface over time [216, 218, 219, 221]. Sol-gel crystalline nanocoatings of calcium phosphate were developed on a variety of substrates [222, 223]. Using calcium phosphate, which is chemically similar to the mineral component of natural bone as a coating, has the added advantage that bioinert implant materials like titanium and cobalt-chromium alloys and alumina can be given bioactive coatings with an improvement of their osseointegration.

Despite the fact that bone-like calcium phosphate nanopowders and nanoplatelets can be synthesized using a variety of production techniques, one very promising approach is to fabricate these materials using a sol-gel solution, which will be discussed in Chapter 13.

Even though biphasic sol-gel HAp products can be produced without difficulties, the results from early studies revealed the syntheses of monophasic calcium phosphate powders and coatings are more challenging. The nanoplatelets and nanoparticles of calcium phosphate provide excellent bioactivity for integration into bone, because of their very high surface areas [216, 218, 219].

11.5. ZIRCONIA

Zirconium dioxide (ZrO_2), or more commonly known as zirconia, is the fully oxidized form of zirconium, and depending on the temperature, it can exist in a number of phases. More importantly, zirconia cannot be manufactured in a pure form owing to certain production issues. Normally, zirconia is stabilized to prevent the formation of cracks. This is the consequence of expansion mismatch caused by structural changes that can take place during heat treatment process. This mismatch may lead to crack formation and fracture of the zirconia ceramic.

The application of zirconia took place after the utilization of alumina as a bioceramic or a biomaterial in general. The word zirconia has been extensively used in the medical field and industry. On the other hand, the zirconia product that is used is in fact partially stabilized zirconia (PSZ), which is a mixture of zirconia with either yttrium trioxide (yttria, Y_2O_3), calcium oxide (calcia, CaO), or magnesium oxide (magnesia, MgO) depending on the synthesis, country of origin, and application. Zirconia and its mixtures has increasingly become a material of choice in implant dentistry, utilized as whole dental implants as well as dental implant abutments [224 - 226].

A small amount of additives can generate partial stabilization which is referred to as partially stabilized zirconia (PSZ). Zirconia, or more appropriately, PSZ-based ceramic material, possesses several advantages which make it a more favorable material as dental implants and in other clinical applications compared to alumina, such as improved corrosion resistance, flexural strength, and fracture toughness which can inhibit crack growth and prevent catastrophic failure [227].

The mechanical properties and durability of zirconia (PSZ) ceramics is strongly influenced by its crystallographic configuration. The crystallographic structures of zirconia are comprised of three different forms. For pure zirconia, the monoclinic phase is stable at room temperature. Zirconia will undergo transformation to a tetragonal phase once it is heated to a temperature between 1170°C and 2360°C. Another phase transformation from a tetragonal phase to a cubic phase will take place when zirconia is heated to a temperature between 2360°C and its melting temperature of 2680°C. The high mechanical properties of zirconia (PSZ) are the result of a toughening mechanism as the ceramic undergoes phase transformation.

Given the fact that the tetragonal and cubic phases of pure zirconia only occur at elevated temperatures, neither of those phases will exist as bulk materials at room temperature. On the other hand, the addition of metallic oxides to zirconia will assist in the stabilization of the phase changes from tetragonal to cubic at low temperature [228]. These metallic oxides include calcia, magnesia, yttria, and cerium trioxide (ceria, Ce_2O_3) [229].

Believed to be utilized as biomedical implants from as early as 1969, zirconia (PSZ) is one of the highest-strength ceramics ideal for biomedical applications [230]. As mentioned earlier, the focus of research has been centered on one type of partially stabilized zirconia known as tetragonal zirconia polycrystal (TZP). Tetragonal zirconia polycrystals are obtained through the addition of metallic oxides such as yttria or ceria to zirconia. More importantly, when yttria is used to stabilize zirconia in comparison to other metallic oxide combinations, mechanical properties can be improved and it is the main type of zirconia currently used for medical purposes [231].

The amount of yttria in TZP only equates to approximately two to three mole percent. An important feature of this yttria stabilized-TZP (Y-TZP) ceramic is its "transformation toughening" effect [230, 231]. The desirable tetragonal phase contains arrays of submicrometer-size grains.

During the transformation of zirconia from tetragonal phase to monoclinic phase, a net volumetric expansion in the ceramic grains will take place, which may place the surface of the zirconia into a compressive stress field that helps it to resist the initiation and progression of cracks. The depth of this residual compressive stress layer has been reported to be several micrometers [232, 233]. The very high strength and fracture toughness of Y-TZP ceramic is based on this "metastability". The Y-TZP ceramic may also transform to the monoclinic phase in an aggressive manner with catastrophic results under more severe environmental conditions of stress and moisture or during certain manufacturing conditions. It is obvious that such a "high metastability" is undesirable for medical implants [230].

11.6. ALUMINA

Aluminum oxide, more commonly referred to as alumina (Al_2O_3), is the most extensively used ceramic oxide material. Alumina ceramics have very high melting or more appropriately dissociation temperature as a result of their strong bonding. Subsequently, the manufacture of alumina ceramics can only be accomplished using high-temperature sintering. The powders are typically heated to two-thirds of their melting temperature during the sintering process. Alumina powder, as a raw material, is produced from the mineral bauxite in large quantities using the Bayer process.

Impurities or additives added will determine the color of alumina. The color can also be governed by the interaction with ionizing radiation and the sintering atmosphere. As a rule in general, alumina is white but can sometimes be pink (88% alumina) or brown (96% alumina) depending on the purity or concentration of alumina. As soon as alumina reacts with chromium oxide (Cr_2O_3), a solid solution is formed and the amount of chromium oxide added will regulate the color of alumina as it changes from white to pink or ruby. Alumina turns white when it is sintered in reducing atmosphere or if it contains traces of silica [234].

Despite the fact that alumina was introduced in the early 1970s for orthopedic applications in France by Boutin and later for dental applications in Germany in 1975, the first recognized requirement for alumina was first published in 1979 by the German Standards' Institute (DIN). This standard was later adopted by the International Standards Organization (ISO) and two more years later still by the American Society for Testing and Materials (ASTM) [203]. The ISO standard was revised in 1994 and this amendment resulted in tougher requirements in terms of bulk density, biaxial flexural strength and grain size. The revised standard also contained a number of additional requirements detailing issues such as compression strength, purity, wear resistance, fatigue strength, and allowed constituents that must be satisfied. A screening test was also included in the ISO standard describing a ring-on-disk test for the wear couple alumina-alumina. The time-consuming simulator testing will be carried out once a material passes this examination. In order to be considered as medical-grade, the alumina ceramic has to pass this test *in vitro* [203].

These standards play a vital role of safeguarding the manufacturing of high-quality ceramic material for use in the biomedical arena. The mechanical, chemical, and physical requirements act as benchmarks for a consistent and high purity product which can be implanted within the human body. These requirements provide specifications for biocompatible grades of alumina to be used in physiological environments.

High-purity alumina has been developed as an alternative to surgical metal alloys for dental and orthopedic applications such as total hip replacement specifically as femoral head and acetabulat components and as early tooth implants (Tubingen implant), and is typically categorized as that with a purity of 99.99% [203].

Medical-grade alumina has a microstructure that consists of a narrow grain-size distribution with a very small grain size of less than seven microns. With the current medical-grade alumina, the average grain size is 1.4 μm and surface finish is normally controlled to a roughness of less than 0.02 μm. Such a microstructure is able of inhibiting static fatigue and slow crack growth while the ceramic is under load.

Furthermore, an excellent surface finish can be easily achieved on alumina ceramic by using a sintering aid such as magnesium oxide (MgO) provided that it contains no porosity and its microstructure is homogeneous and consists of small fine grains. The amount of sintering additives found in medical-grade alumina is extremely low with a typical concentration of less than 0.5 wt.%. Nonetheless, process such as hot isostatic pressing can be used to improve the microstructure and the density of the bioceramic. Corundum (α-Al_2O_3) is the phase associated with medical-grade alumina and it is known to be a very stable phase.

On the other hand, alumina suffers from a fundamental flaw when used as an implant material for dental and orthopedic applications. This is due to the fact that a non-adherent fibrous membrane may develop at the bone-implant interface similar to other "inert" biomaterials (Fig. **35**). This can be avoided by modifying the alumina surface or using it directly in articulating area such as in a knee or hip prosthesis. Under certain conditions, interfacial failure can occur resulting in the loosening of the implant. This was observed in some earlier dental implant designs.

The excellent corrosion resistance, high hardness, and low coefficient of friction of alumina offer a very low rate of wear when it is used as an articulating surface in orthopedic applications. The mechanical behavior of alumina ceramics under simulated physiological environments has led to long-term survival predictions while exposed to sub-critical stresses. The stress magnitude of medical-grade alumina was projected to be 112 MPa for a 50-year period with a 99.9% survival probability [203].

Other applications for alumina in orthopedic and maxillofacial applications include femoral head components, alumina stems, alumina spacers employed specifically in revision surgery [235] and ceramic knee prostheses. Furthermore, alumina in single crystal (Bioceram) and polycrystalline forms has been previously used in dental applications as tooth implants [208, 236 - 238].

As discussed in the previous section, partially stabilized zirconia (PSZ) in addition to alumina has been accepted as a ceramic material for use in clinical applications. Despite the fact that both ceramic materials are effective, they have specific potential drawbacks. Alumina, for example, is a brittle material with a risk of fracture even though it exhibits excellent wear properties and hardness. This hard but brittle property combination means that certain design restrictions apply. On the other hand, the hardness of PSZ is only half of that of alumina but its fracture resistance can be improved through transformation toughening. As a result, its overall bending strength and toughness are substantially much higher than those of alumina. Subsequently, an ideal material would be a ceramic that combines the best properties of alumina and zirconia. This leads to the new generation of ceramics referred to as zirconia-toughened alumina.

The improvements in toughness and strength of zirconia-toughened alumina can be attributed to the stress-induced transformation-toughening mechanism created by the presence of fine zirconia particles in suitable quantities and distributed all through the alumina body. Hypothetically, it is due to the transformation-toughening theory given that the crystal structure of the zirconia particles in the region of the crack will transform to the stable monoclinic phase from the metastable tetragonal phase as a crack grows through the ceramic. This phase change is expected to increase the volume of the particles by about 3 to 4%. This volume change also creates compressive stresses within the alumina matrix. These stresses in turn close the crack and serve as an energy barrier to prevent additional crack growth. The incorporation of zirconia to the alumina matrix was initiated to improve fracture toughness and strength. Yet, long-term clinical studies are necessary in order to demonstrate its effectiveness as a new- generation high-performance material [203].

In 2002, a new batch-processed zirconia-toughened alumina ceramic was developed by Insley *et al.* [239]. The new zirconia-toughened alumina ceramic consists of 75% alumina and 25% zirconia with no presence of mixed oxides. In terms of mechanical properties, the new zirconia-toughened alumina possesses a significantly lower flexural strength in comparison to commercially available zirconia-toughened alumina ceramics such as Biolox® Delta. As explained by Insley *et al.* [239], the main reason for this difference in the mechanical properties is due to the coarser grain size within the microstructure of their ceramic. In addition to the grain size, the distribution of the zirconia grains within the alumina matrix is also dissimilar. Again, long-term clinical studies are essential to prove its effectiveness as a better new-generation high-performance biomaterial.

11.7. BIOACTIVE GLASS

Various types of bioactive glasses and glass ceramics have been developed ever since their discovery in the 1960s by Hench and co-workers. Given the fact that they can bond to living tissues (Bioglass®) and their unique properties such as high machinability and fast setting ability can be tailored simply by manipulating the morphology and compositions, many clinical Bioglass® and other similar compositions and structures are being employed in dental and maxillofacial surgery as well as for orthopedics for bone augmentation and restoration, and in the field of tissue engineering in general [240].

As one of the vital trace elements within the human body, silicon (Si) are found at a level of 100 ppm in the bone and 200-550 ppm bound to extracellular matrix compounds [216]. The location of silicon was discovered to be at active calcification sites in the bones and contributes to the mineralization process of bone growth [217]. Interestingly, a study has demonstrated that the growth of dental pulp stem cells were encouraged on silicon scaffolds functionalized with (3-Aminopropyl) Trimethoxysilane (APTMS)/toluene, suggesting that it could potentially be used in tissue engineering applications [241].

Stimulated by the silicon function in human body, the behavior of stem cells on silicon nanoporous and mesoporous matrices, and the bioactive compositions of silicate-based bioglass, a new family of bioactive calcium silicate ceramics has been created during the past decade with various compositions. It was discovered that bioactive silicate ceramics with specific compositions could significantly promote *in vitro* osteogenic differentiation for several stem cells and *in vivo* osteogenesis and angiogenesis.

Glasses that are mainly based on silica (SiO_2) that may also contain small amounts of other crystalline phases have been investigated for implantation purposes [242]. The compositions of the first-generation bioactive glass fall within the Na_2O-CaO-P_2O_5-SiO_2 system. First proposed in 1971, a bioglass called 45S5 Bioglass®

with a composition of 42% SiO_2, 24.5% CaO, 24.5% Na_2O, and 6% P_2O_5 by weight was developed [243], and it was suggested that this bioglass has greater osteoblastic activity which is attributed to a rapid exchange of alkali ions with hydronium ions at the surface compared to hydroxyapatite (HAp) [235, 244]. This in turn leads to the formation of a silica-rich layer over a period of time. The migration of calcium (Ca^{2+}) and phosphate (PO_4^{3+}) ions are permitted on this layer to the silica-rich surface where they combined with soluble Ca^{2+} and PO_4^{3+} ions from the solution. This results in the formation of an amorphous CaO-P_2O_5 layer. This layer will then undergo crystallization upon interacting with hydroxide (OH), carbonate (CO_3^{2+}) and fluoride (F) ions from solution. A similar phenomenon was also observed in a number of studies in bioglass with slightly modified compositions [242, 245].

Furthermore, the formation of an apatite layer was observed in glass ceramics with a similar composition and various degrees of crystallinity [246]. It was suggested that the formation of this layer was directly influenced by the amount of glassy phase that still remains and the formation ceases once the glassy phase constitutes less than approximately 5 wt.%.

Bioactive glass with precipitated crystalline apatite and reduced alkaline oxide content can be produced through the application of a specific heat treatment technique. The resultant glass ceramic is known as Ceravitals. In comparison to Bioglass®, Creavitals possesses greater mechanical strength but reduced bioactivity.

A glass ceramic comprised of Oxyfluorapatite ($Ca_{10}(PO_4)_6(OH,F_2)$) and wollastonite ($CaO \cdot SiO_2$) in an MgO-CaO-SiO_2 glassy matrix was produced by Kokubo *et al.* [247] and it is known as A-W glass ceramic (Cerabone A-W). It was reported in the early 1990s that the A-W glass ceramic spontaneously bonded to living bone without the formation of fibrous tissue around the glass. Moreover, a machinable bioactive glass ceramic composed of apatite and phlogophite ($(Na,K)Mg_3(Al-Si_3O_{10})(F)_2$) called Bioverits was also developed and was previously used as artificial vertebra [247]. In spite of this, its current production and application are restricted only to research and the commercial production of A-W glass has been discontinued.

11.7.1. Glass-to-Bone: Bonding

Bioactive glasses with a certain compositional range containing CaO, SiO_2, P_2O_5, and Na_2O and in specific proportions have shown to display proper glass-to-bone bonding. Compared to commercial soda-lime-silica glasses, there are three compositional variations separating it from bioactive glass. These variations include a SiO_2 content of less than 60%, a high Na_2O and CaO content, and a high

CaO/P_2O_5 ratio. As a result of these compositional features, highly reactive surfaces are created after the bioactive glass is exposed to an aqueous medium.

On the other hand, given the amount of silica found in bioactive glasses ranging between 45 to 60%, problems associated with the formation of phase separation and crystallization of the glassy material can easily become an issue as a consequence of repeated hot working process [243, 248]. The crystallization of the glass can lead to a decrease in the rate of bioactivity [249], and a glassy phase of incontrollable composition is the outcome of partial crystallization. Nevertheless, crystallization can be controlled by using the chemical composition of the bioactive glass [250].

A new generation of bioactive glasses in the $Na_2O-K_2O-MgO-CaO-B_2O_3-P_2O_5-SiO_2$ system has been shown to display the capacity to be heated repeatedly without the risk of devitrification [251]. Microspheres can therefore be produced and sintered into porous implants of various sizes and shapes [252]. The porosity of a bioactive glass body can significantly increase the total amount of surface area available for interaction between glass and bone, and this in turn will permit the formation of a three-dimensional healing bony tissue. Through the utilizations of various sintering times and temperatures, the mechanical strength and porosity of the bioactive glass implant can be manipulated [253]. In order to attain the best mechanical strength of the sintered implant, the glass must retain its amorphous structure throughout the heat treatment process.

11.7.2. Glass-to-Bone: Interfacial Bond Strength

The same conclusion has been reached in a number of studies that due to the interfacial chemical reactions on the surface of bioactive glass, a firm and unique bonding is achieved between the glass implant and human bone. The strength of this bonding has been demonstrated using mechanical testing by determining the push-out to failure force. The interfacial strength obtained can then be used to compare the performance of different biomaterials.

A firm layer of calcium phosphate was identified in a previous study as the true bond between bioactive glasses and host bone tissue [249]. In spite of this, the study also revealed that only a low interfacial strength is reached when aluminum (Al^{3+}) of approximately 42.5 wt.% is added to glasses containing approximately 60 wt.% SiO_2. Furthermore, no bone contact is achieved at all for glass containing both SiO_2 and Al^{3+} with amounts greater than 60 wt.% and 2.5 wt.%, respectively. The study also discovered that the bonding strength of titanium implants (when used as reference) was only about one-tenth of the strength achieved using bioactive glass implants.

A similar difference in the bond strength between titanium and bioactive glass implants was also observed in another study that utilizes the same testing approach [254]. The bonding of bioactive glass to bone was hypothesized to be based on the formation of a calcium phosphate layer connecting the bioglass implant to the host bone and an even dissolution of material. This hypothesis can be verified by evaluating the bond strength of implants made from bioactive glass and HAp [254 - 256].

Interfacial bond strength has been found to differ between different materials due to their structure, composition, and morphology. These findings also support the notion of separating bioactive materials in two distinct groups based on their bioactivity. Hypothetically, the silica-rich gel is the weakest point of the interface between bioactive glass and bone. On the other hand, the results of push-out failure by the maximum force according to mechanical testing in most cases occur by fracture of the bone in close proximity to the glass implant [257, 258].

As previously discussed, the ability to firmly bond to bone *via* chemical reactions is an important asset of bioactive glasses. Eventually, this permits the glass to be replaced by bone and this makes it ideal for use in medical applications. More importantly, the elements found in bioactive glass are physiological chemicals or minerals discovered in the body such as calcium, phosphorus, silicon, oxygen, potassium, magnesium, and sodium. It has been reported that the concentration of the specific elements never increases to a level that could disturb the adjacent tissues during the bonding and formation of bone [257, 259]. However, the mechanical properties of glass restrict the use of bioactive glass as an implant material or in the manufacturing of medical devices.

The brittle nature or glass subsequently means that it cannot be utilized in situations where load-bearing properties are essential. Glass can be molded into rods and plates. It can also be manufactured into rigid medical devices by grinding and cutting cast rods. They can also be employed as filler materials in the form of particulates. Another possibility that has been extensively investigated is a bioactive coating produced from bioactive glass on mechanically tougher implant materials.

11.7.3. Bioactivity of the Glass

As discussed above, the rates of osteostimulation between different types of bioactive particulates have been determined in a study by Oonishi *et al.* and this provided the fundamental *in vivo* assessments concerning Class A and Class B bioactive materials [260].

For Class A bioactive glasses, soluble silicic acid is rapidly released, followed by calcium ions (Ca^{2+}). This in turn leads to a quicker precipitation of calcium phosphate on the depleted Si-rich glass surface.

On the other hand, Class B bioactive glasses possess a low network dissolution rate [261, 262]. Glasses containing less than 55 wt.% SiO_2 have a high rate of dissolution [262]. It has been shown that a higher concentration of SiO_2 in the glass will result in a lower rate of network dissolution and formation of a Si-rich layer. Once the concentration of SiO_2 in glass exceeds about 60 wt.%, the rate of Si-rich gel formation on the glass surface is so low that it has no practical significance on the bioactivity.

A reasonable mechanism was first suggested by Strnad [263] and later by Karlsson and Ylänen [264] as they discovered that the bioactivity of glass is founded on the mean number of non-bridging oxygen ions in the silica tetrahedron. The charge of the oxygen ion in the corner of the tetrahedron is balanced by a network modifier anion which is Na^+, K^+ or Ca^{2+} instead of sharing a corner with another tetrahedron. As a result of rapid exchanges between these anions for H^+ or H_3O^+ from the solution which occurs once exposed to body fluid, a hydration of the gel structure (= Si-(OH)) instead of (=Si-O Na^+, K^+) occurs.

Each silicon in silicate glasses is bonded to four oxygen atoms. Therefore, the number of non-bridging oxygen ions in the tetrahedron can be of any value between zero and four. If the number is zero, it signifies a fully polymerized, three-dimensional network of silica tetrahedral. However, when the number is four, it indicates a dissolved SiO_4 ion. The number must be greater than 2.6 in order to achieve bioactivity for a glass with a SiO_2 content of less than 60 wt.% (Table **13**).

Table 13. The number of non-bridging oxygen ions as a function of wt.% of SiO_2 and Na_2O content in a glass [242].

Q^n	Non-Bridging Oxygen Ions	SiO_2	Na_2O
0	4	33.3	66.6
1	3	40	60
2	2	50	50
3	1	66.6	33.3
4	0	100	0

Two to three non-bridging oxygen ions will result as soon as the concentrations of SiO_2 on the surfaces of glasses reach between 50 and 55 wt.%. This causes hydration of two or three oxygen ions with each silica tetrahedron, forming ¼·Si(OH)$_2$ or -Si(OH)$_3$. The relationship between the role of non-bridging oxygen ions and the bioactivity of the glass was examined in studies by Serra *et al.* [265, 266].

The silica network is broken partially during dissolution of the glass and the SiOH and Si(OH)$_4$ groups are located on the uppermost layer of the glass. The higher the number of non-bridging oxygen ions in the gel, the higher the bioactivity of the glass. If none of the four oxygen ions is bridged, then a totally dissolved monomeric SiO$_4$ ion will form during the final stages. In this case, the concentration of SiO$_2$ will need to be very low, for example less than 40 wt.%. Questions arise as to whether or not it is possible to obtain a glass phase of this composition [267]. The crucial factor controlling the bioactivity of a glass is said to be the formation of the hydrated Si-rich gel on the glass surface for which the SiO$_2$ content should be 50 to 60 wt.%.

11.7.4. Bioactive Glass: Production Method

Bioactive glasses have been produced using conventional glass manufacturing techniques. The carbonates and oxide components of glass in the form of grains are mixed, melted and then homogenized at a temperature between 1250 and 1400°C [268]. Bulk implants are manufactured by casting molten glass into graphite or steel molds. In order to achieve the required tolerances, a final grind and polish is sometimes necessary. By producing different particle sizes directly, this process has a number of advantages despite the fact that the method has been modified a number of times so that grinding and polishing can be avoided.

Nanoscale bioactive glasses have been produced using various approaches such as sol-gel and flame spray synthesis. The availability of nanoparticles and nanofibers of bioactive glass more than a few years ago resulted in their use in the biomedical arena as a nanocomposite with and without the addition of polymers.

11.7.4.1. Flame Spray or Gas Phase Synthesis of Glass Nanoparticles

At the moment, one of the techniques used to prepare nanoparticles are based on heating metal-organic precursor compounds at temperatures above 1000°C *via* flame spray technology. Another commonly used technique is spray drying. While flame spray technique is an energy-intensive approach, its advantage lies in the fact that additional energy is not needed for the precursors compared to other gas phase techniques.

The basic principle behind all gas phase synthesis approach involves the formation of molecular nuclei followed by condensation and coalescence. During the process, this induces the subsequent growth of nanoparticles in high-temperature regions [269, 270].

In an attempt to gain a deeper understanding of the dynamics and key variables of flame spray process and how they can be controlled in order to obtain nanoparticles of given size range and chemical composition, a number of studies were carried out and it was discovered that the metal-carboxylate system is an extremely convenient precursor because it allows for the synthesis of oxide nanoparticles of virtually any composition [271, 272]. Most importantly, metal-organic frameworks are fully miscible among each other and can tolerate humidity. They are also highly stable in air. Consequently, the fabrication of nanoparticulate mixed oxides of different types with high chemical homogeneity is permitted using this process.

Utilizing the flame spray process, bioactive glass nanoparticles with diameters ranging between 20 to 50 nm have been synthesized and it was reported that a pronounced increase in mineral content was observed when human dentin was treated with these nanoparticles, suggesting rapid remineralization [273]. In a later study, the capability of flame spray technique to synthesize radio-opaque bioactive glass nanoparticles was also demonstrated for potential use in root canal applications [274].

11.7.4.2. Laser Spinning Technique

Laser spinning technique has been demonstrated to be an efficient method for synthesizing bioactive glass nanofibers. Nanostructures of bioactive glasses can also be produced with potential applications in tissue engineering as scaffolds and as fillers in bone defects. They can also be used as reinforcing agents in the manufacturing of nanocomposites.

The potential to create nanofibers with different rates of bioresorption using laser spinning technique is evident by its capacity to produce nanofibers with a wide range of compositions. The changes in the rate of bioresorption can then be used to control the release of active ions that have the potential to stimulate the gene expression and cellular response necessary for tissue regeneration [275, 276].

One of the advantages of laser spinning technique is its speed as the process is relatively fast and the nanofibers can be manufactured within several microseconds. Another advantage is its ability to synthesize glass nanofibers of compositions that would be challenging to obtain using other techniques. The diameters of the fibers produced using the laser spinning technique varies from hundreds down to tenths of microns. Furthermore, the types of products can range from disordered mats to continuous filaments [277]. However, the major drawback of laser spinning is that high energy is required during the fabrication process, which resulted in an increase in production costs.

11.7.4.3. Micro-Emulsions

By definition, micro-emulsions in many cases are thermodynamically stable dispersions of oil and water stabilized by a surfactant and a co-surfactant. Micro-emulsions can be of the droplet type, either with spherical water droplets dispersed in a continuous medium of oil or vice versa with spherical oil droplets dispersed in a continuous medium of water. Studies have discovered that nanoparticle size and polydispersity can be regulated simply by adjusting the micro-emulsion as well as other operation variables [278, 279].

It has been well known that this method is ideal for obtaining nanometer-sized inorganic particles with minimum agglomeration [280, 281]. The major drawbacks with the micro-emulsion approach are its low yield in production as well as the need for a large quantity of oil and surfactant phases. Very few studies are currently available that describes the production of nanosized bioactive particles using micro-emulsion technique despite the fact that it offers a different approach for synthesizing many forms of organic and inorganic nanometer-sized particles compared to other production methods [282, 283].

11.7.4.4. Sol-Gel

Compared to traditional glass melting or ceramic powder methods, the advantage associated with sol-gel processing is above all the potential to achieve higher purity and homogeneity in addition to the lower processing temperatures accompanying with the approach [284].

Using the sol-gel process, the production of bioglass and other ceramics has become an interesting research field over the past four decades [284 - 289]. Bioactive glasses can be synthesized by sintering gels at temperatures between 600 and 700°C. This eliminates most of the disadvantages of high temperature processing with much better control over purity. In addition, a broader range and better control of bioactivity can be achieved by either changing the composition or microstructure through processing parameters [290].

It has been suggested that the high bioactivity of sol-gel derived materials is related to the microstructural features of the gel. These features include pore and grain sizes associated with the large surface area, and higher rate of dissolution and negative surface charge [291]. Consequently, sol-gel derived bioactive glass has been suggested as an alternative to glasses that are synthesized through melt and quenching methods based on their ability to exhibit excellent degradation and/or resorption properties, improved homogeneity and purity, more rapid bone bonding, and higher rate of apatite layer formation [268].

11.7.4.5. Bioactive Glass Composites

The rationale behind the development of bioactive glass composites is to optimize and combine the bioactive phase of glass fibers or particles with the exceptional mechanical properties of metals or polymers to enhance properties such as flexibility and the ability to withstand deformation under loading. A number of bioglass composites have been developed and investigated for biomedical applications such as dental implant, drug delivery systems, and as bone regeneration matrix and scaffolds [242].

11.7.5. Biomedical Applications

As a result of their surface activity, bioactive glasses including Bioglass® are being used for bone augmentation and restoration, in orthopedics, dental and maxillofacial surgery and in the field of tissue engineering. They have proved to be efficient, some even out performing other bioceramic and metal prostheses [242].

11.7.5.1. Treatment of Dentin Hypersensitivity

During the past decade, a number of consumer and professional products containing bioactive glass have been introduced into the market (45S5 Bioglass®). Oravive®, which is a daily use fluoride-free dentifrice, was the first product developed by NovaMin® Technologies that contains 5% of the bioactive glass ingredient NovaMin®. This product was cleared for use by FDA through a 510(k) product as a medical device for the rapid and continual reduction of tooth sensitivity through physical tubule occlusion. At present, CSPS has been formulated into over 15 products and is sold in over 20 countries, including the USA, Canada, India, China, and a number of countries in Europe. These products have proven to be highly effective and the CSPS material has an unparalleled safety profile [242].

A new and improved bioglass toothpaste formulation called BioMin has been developed by researchers. In addition to addressing tooth sensitivity, the makers of BioMin claimed that the toothpaste could also aid in the prevention of tooth decay and acid erosion. This is due to the capacity of the bioglass to form a protective enamel-mimicking layer and slowly releasing fluoride into the mouth. Sensodyne Repair and Protect, manufactured by GlaxoSmithKline (GSK), is an over-the-counter dentifrice that provides NovaMin® technology to the consumer in many parts of the world [292].

11.7.5.2. Maxillofacial and Ear, Nose, and Throat

Porous and rigid bioactive glass bodies can be manufactured by sintering bioactive glass microspheres. The rate of bone ingrowth into the three-dimensional porosity network within the bioactive glass material is significantly higher in comparison to porous titanium with similar porosity [293].

In the treatment of profound deafness, a number of electronic components are utilized within appropriate devices, and the electrodes attached to these electronic devices are coated with Bioglass® before the device is placed on the inner and outer of the middle ear [294]. A firm anchoring is achieved once the device is inserted and the part is exposed to bone. The other part of the bioactive glass-coated anchor passes through the eardrum and bonds to the soft tissue, thereby providing a seal between the inner and outer ear.

Bioglass® in the form of cone-shaped implants has been used to fill or replace defects in the mandible and maxilla as well as small bones in the middle ear. The glass also displays the ability to bond to soft tissues, which has created new possibilities for wider medical applications in ear, throat, and nose surgery. However, findings from studies by Stoor *et al.* [295 - 297] suggested that the promising results supporting the use of bioactive glass material in ear, nose, and throat surgery are limited as a consequence of the antibacterial effects of bioactive glass paste on oral microorganisms and bacterial infections [297].

Solid-shaped bioactive glasses of various compositions such as S53P4 were also used to replace the bone structure that supports the eye as well as in the treatment of facial injuries [298, 299]. The results of a clinical trial suggested that using thin and slowly resorbable bioactive glass would provide a promising option for the reconstruction of orbital floor defects. Table **14** shows the composition differences between Bioglass® and S53P4, both of which have been widely used for clinical applications.

Table 14. Composition variations between Bioglass® and S53P4 [242].

	Elements			
	SiO_2	Na_2O	CaO	P_2O_5
Bioglass®	45	24.5	24.5	6
S53P4	53	23	20	4

In an effort to prevent resorption after tooth extraction, the concept of filling the hole in the mandible using bioglass was proposed [300]. In their study, conical implants were fabricated using injection molding. A mating drill bit is used to prepare the bone for the implant to achieve the best possible fit of the conical implant. In addition, bioactive glass particles are widely used in odontology to fill defects associated with periodontal disease, such as the loss of bone that surrounds the tooth [301].

CHAPTER 12

Bone Tissue Engineering and Scaffolds

Abstract: Tissue engineering in recent years has taken a new direction by seizing the advantage of combining the use of living cells with three-dimensional ceramic scaffolds to deliver vital cells to the damaged site of the patient. Productive and feasible strategies have been initiated during the last few decades to combine bioceramic implants with biogenic materials to the field of cell growth and differentiation of osteogenic cells. The reconstruction of bone tissue utilizing nanocomposite bone grafts with composition, biomechanical, biological, physiochemical and structural features that mimic those of natural bone is an objective to be pursued.

Keywords: Bioactive glass, Bioceramics, Bioglass, Bone regeneration, Calcium phosphate, Coralline apatite, Glass ceramics, Hydroxyapatite HAp, Liposomes, Nanobioceramics, Nanocomposites.

Long ago, the focus of bone tissue engineering has been undeniably centered on the modifications in materials and nanotechnology. Although the addition of material requirements is normal during the design and development of engineered bone substitutes, of vital importance is the inclusion of clinical prerequisites so that clinically relevant devices and prosthetics can be engineered.

At present, the emphasis of tissue engineering has changed by seizing the advantage of combining the use of living cells with three-dimensional ceramic scaffolds to transport vital cells to the damaged site of the patient. Productive and feasible strategies have been initiated during the last few decades to combine bioceramic implants with biogenic materials to the arena of cell growth and differentiation of osteogenic cells.

A number of clinical arguments exist related to the advancement of bone tissue-engineering substitutes, including a need for better filler materials during the reconstruction of large bone defects, and for implants which are more mechanically suited to their biological surroundings. From a biological perspective, the traditional methods used in the management of bone defects include autografting and allografting.

Andy H. Choi and Besim Ben-Nissan

Four components are required for bone regeneration [302 - 304]:

1. A morphogenetic signal;
2. Responsive host cells that will react to the signal;
3. A carrier of this signal that is suitable and capable of transporting it to specific sites. This carrier also has to function as scaffolding to cater for the growth of responsive host cells; and
4. Most importantly, a viable and well-vascularized host bed.

A scaffolding material is employed either to serve as a carrier or template for implanted bone cells or other agents, or to induce the formation of bone from the surrounding tissue. A composite scaffold that combines a polymer with a bioceramic would ideally unite the advantages of the two materials where the polymer would improve the toughness of the composite and the bioceramic would increase the bioactivity of the resulting composite. The concept of a polymer ceramic composite with enhanced fracture resistance was investigated in a study by Peroglio *et al.* [305]. Polycaprolactone (PCL)-coated alumina scaffolds were produced and characterized. Alumina scaffolds were sintered utilizing a foam replication approach, and the polymer coating was attained by diffusing the scaffold with either a PCL solution or nanodispersion.

The progression of bone regeneration is normal in the repair of fractures. The stages involved in the remodeling cycle include the introduction of bone grafts, the skeletal homeostasis and the cascading sequence of biological events.

A stem cell is a cell from an embryo, foetus or adult which has the capability to reproduce for long periods. It can also give rise to specialized cells that make up the tissues and organs of the body. It has been demonstrated that these cells when implanted into immuno-deficient mice can algamate with mineralized three-dimensional scaffolds to create highly vascularized bone tissues. Defects across the bone diaphysis can be treated with these cell cultured-bioceramic composites with good functional recovery and exceptional integration between bone tissue and ceramic scaffold. Significant innovative works with nanobioceramics are in progress and medical applications are becoming quite common.

Utilizing nanocomposite bone grafts to reconstruct bone tissue with features such as physiochemical, biological, structural, biomechanical, and compositional which imitates those of natural bone is an objective worthy of pursuing. It is a recognized fact that natural bone is composed of nanosized and plate-like crystals of HAp grown in close contact with an organic matrix that is rich in collagen fibers. Using strategies discovered in nature is one novel approach in the fabrication of nanocomposite bone grafts that have received much attention in recent times and this approach is perceived to be advantageous compared to conventional techniques.

12.1. CALCIUM PHOSPHATE

A calcium compound, tri-calcium phosphate, was first used in the early 1900's in bone repair with great success [306]. However, it took more than six decades after the first clinical study by Hulbert *et al.* [307] that a proposal was made regarding the use of porous calcium phosphate scaffolds in the treatment of bone defects. The motivation driving the exploration and development of biomaterials based on calcium phosphate for bone augmentation, substitution, and repair was attributable to the close resemblance in composition between synthetic and biological apatites [308].

During the past two decades, significant devotion has also been paid to bioactive composite grafts that are composed of bioactive ceramic filler such as calcium phosphate in a polymeric matrix. In essence, these bioactive composite grafts are intended to attain interfacial bonding between the graft and host tissues. The most notable examples of bioactive composite grafts include calcium phosphate-polyethylene, calcium phosphate-Ti-6Al-4V and calcium phosphate-collagen [309, 310]. A number of production approaches have been utilized in the manufacture of collagen-calcium phosphate composite films, gels, collagen-coated ceramics, ceramic-coated collagen matrices and composite scaffolds for hard tissue repair [311].

The potential application of high-density polyethylene in combination with calcium phosphate nanoparticles as scaffolds was explored in a study by Hild *et al.* [312]. The lack of cytotoxic effects of the scaffolds was confirmed by viability assays. After haematoxylin and eosin staining, microscopic images also demonstrated typical growth and morphology.

A natural choice for bone grafting and of particular interest is the calcium phosphate-collagen composite graft [313]. Skeletal bones are mainly composed of collagen and carbonate-substituted hydroxyapatite, both of which are osteoconductive components. Hence, an implant produced using calcium phosphate and collagen is expected to behave in a similar manner. In addition, a composite of collagen and calcium phosphate has been shown to be biocompatible in both humans and animals [314].

In comparison to monolithic calcium phosphate, a composite matrix displayed better osteoconductive properties once human-like osteoblast cells are embedded, which also induces the production of calcification of an identical bone matrix. Furthermore, collagen-calcium phosphate composites have proven to mechanically behave in a superior fashion compared to the collagen and calcium phosphate individually. The ductile properties of collagen helped to improve the poor fracture toughness of calcium phosphates.

The application of nano-HAp-tricalcium phosphate biphasic composites was proposed in a study by Ebrahimi *et al.* [315] based on the works of Daculsi *et al.* [316] and LeGeros *et al.* [317, 318], and that the simple addition of collagen may improve the physical properties of biphasic calcium phosphate scaffolds while enhancing their bioactivity. After sintering, the dimensional shrinkage of large scaffolds was discovered to be lesser than small scaffolds. Furthermore, scaffolds with high nano-HAp ratios suffered greater dimensional changes in comparison to those with high β-tricalcium phosphate ratios.

A range of biodegradable synthetic and natural polymers have been suggested and explored in combination with calcium phosphate as scaffolding materials for tissue engineering applications [311, 319]. Synthetic polymers contain many advantages, for example, their physical-chemical properties can be altered and the degradation and mechanical characteristics can be engineered to meet the desired requirements simply by changing the chemical composition. Another advantage synthetic polymers possess is their ability to be bioactivated with specific molecules through the combinations of side chains and functional groups.

Regarded as one of the most widely employed biodegradable polymer which can be easily processed, the application of poly(lactic-*co*-glycolic acid) or PLGA has unfortunately been severely restricted due to its hydrophobic surface, poor bioactivity, and weak mechanical strength. In light of the biodegradable and biocompatible nature of polymers such as PLGA and the structural and physiochemical benefits of nano-calcium phosphate in the formation of new bone, a composite composed of PLGA and nano-calcium phosphate has been hypothesized and considered as a solution in regulating the adhesion and the osteogenic differentiation of human mesenchymal stem cells (hMSCs) [320, 321]. Using avian vessels from the chick chorioallantoicmembrane, the *in vivo* behavior of an electrospun nanocomposite composed of amorphous calcium phosphate nanoparticles and PLGA seeded with human adipose-derived stem cells was confirmed in a study which has completely infiltrated the nanocomposite within one week [322].

It has been suggested that the use of polyamide with its high toughness could improve the brittle nature of nano-calcium phosphate in applications such as the reconstruction of bone defects in the mandible [323, 324]. An *in vivo* study using rabbit models revealed the amount of new bone formed around the composite was found to be substantial at marrow-rich implantation sites, but bone marrow stromal cells (BMSCs) was required at marrow-poor sites. A similar observation was recorded in their *in vitro* investigation where the composite stimulated the expression of osteogenic proteins and displayed excellent secretion of active alkaline phosphatase and bioactivity with considerable BMSC proliferation [323].

To improve the biocompatibility and mechanical properties, an investigation was carried out to investigate the feasibility of utilizing gelatin in combination with calcium phosphate and polycaprolactone (PCL) for the manufacture of nanocomposite scaffolds. In a study, the *in vitro* and *in vivo* behavior of the composite seeded with dental pulp stem cells (DPSCs) was examined [325]. Histological evaluation revealed that the implants were covered by a thin fibrous tissue capsule without any adverse effects but no sign of tissue ingrowth after the scaffolds seeded with DPSCs were subcutaneously inserted into immuno-compromised nude mice.

A new approach to alleviate dentine hypersensitivity was attempted through the specific engineered regeneration of enamel [326]. Electrospun mats of amorphous calcium phosphate/poly(vinylpyrrolidone) micro- and nano-fibers were synthesized and served as hydrogel mats that direct and promote *in vitro* remineralization of dental enamel in the presence of fluoride. The procedure resulted in the *in situ* transformation of spherical amorphous calcium phosphate phase at the surface of the enamel to generate a contiguous overlayer of crystalline fluoridated hydroxyapatite with a thickness of approximately 500 nm after one hour of treatment. The study hypothesized that the electrospun mats can be utilized as high-concentration reservoirs of amorphous calcium phosphate for the remineralization of acid-etched dental enamel and occlusion of exposed dentinal tubules *in vitro*.

12.1.1. Nanocoated Coralline Apatite

At present, a number of natural and synthetic bone-graft materials in use are synthesized from coralline HAp. Commercial coralline HAp, as a consequence of their conversion process, has retained coral or $CaCO_3$ and the structure retains nanopores within the inter-pore trabeculae, giving rise to high rates of dissolution.

Under specific circumstances, there characteristics reduced the strength and durability of the coralline HAp and making them impossible to be used in applications where high structural strength is essential. To overcome these restrictions, a double- stage conversion approach was created, and the method is comprised of two different stages. During the first step, a complete conversion of coral to 100% calcium phosphate is achieved. In the second step, a sol-gel-derived calcium phosphate nanocoating is applied directly to cover the meso- and nanopores within the intra-pore material, while maintaining the large pores [218,

219].

Mechanical properties such as elastic modulus and fracture toughness, as well as biaxial and compression strengths were respectively enhanced as a consequence of this novel double-stage treatment process. More importantly, this treatment process is anticipated to enhance the bioactivity as a result of the nanograin size and thus large surface area which enhances the reactivity of the nanocoating. It is expected that this material could be used in bone-graft applications in which high-strength and load-bearing requirements are vital.

12.1.2. Liposomes

Considered as one of the most clinically established nanoscale systems currently used in the delivery of non-toxic and antifungal drugs, genes, and vaccines, liposomes consist of a single layer, or multiple concentric lipid bilayers, that encapsulate an aqueous compartment. Due to their excellent biocompatibility, the combination of calcium phosphate and liposome has shown great potential as candidates for bone regeneration [327, 328].

Liposome-coated HAp and tricalcium phosphate were first used in the late 1990s as bone implants for the treatment of mandibular bony defect in miniature swine [327]. Artificial bony defects on one side acted as controls, whilst defects on the other side were either implanted with tricalcium phosphate-coated or HAp-coated liposomes. Histology and radiography were performed at three weeks and six weeks after surgery. The implant material was covered by dense connective tissues after three weeks, while new bone formation was noticeable near the implanted material after six weeks.

In another study, a 1.2 cm-diameter bone defect created on rabbit cranium was treated with the bone morphogenetic protein-2 gene (cDNA plasmid) introduced with porous calcium phosphate after completion of hemostasis, and the influence of using cationic liposomes as a vector to the amounts of new bone formation was investigated [328]. It was observed that even though the formation of new bone was obvious surrounding the scaffold three weeks post-operation, the induced bone tissue did not occupy all the pores of the scaffold even at nine weeks post-operation.

12.2. BIOGLASS

As discussed earlier, bioactive glasses have been used successfully in clinical situation as bone-filling materials [329 - 331]. A 3-D bioactive scaffold with hierarchical interconnected pore morphologies similar to trabecular bone was developed using sol-gel derived bioactive glasses and its potential to fulfill the criteria for an ideal scaffold for bone tissue engineering has been assessed in a study [332]. Possessing the minimum pore diameter vital for tissue ingrowth and vascularization in the human body, the scaffolds comprise of a pore network with macropores greater than 500 μm that are connected by pore windows with diameters greater than 100 μm. In addition, the scaffolds also contain textural porosity in the mesopore range, which is between 10 to 20 nm. The compressive strength reported was in close proximity to that of trabecular bone.

The tensile bending strength for many bioactive glass compositions is in the range of 40 and 60 MPa. They also have a low elastic modulus of between 30 and 35 GPa.

Despite the fact that studies conducted on the applications of bioactive glass as bone grafts focused mainly on orthopedic applications and on areas such as the femur, the same principle can be used in oral and maxillofacial applications.

The histological sequence of osteostimulation by 45S5 Bioglass® particulate was measured using a critical-size defect model in a rabbit femoral condyle [260]. The studies on bioglass showed that bone formation is more rapid in the presence of the osteostimulation particles coupled with the regeneration of a more highly mineralized quality of bone in the defect compared to synthetic calcium phosphate particles. The rate of bone regeneration in the Oonishi model is connected to the release rate of the soluble silicon and calcium ions from the particulates investigated. For rapid bone regeneration, a quick release rate is crucial and the defect should be filled ideally by the regenerated trabecular bone tissue.

Solid-shaped bioactive glass implants have been examined for the reconstruction of deep osteochondral defects using animal models [333 - 335]. The findings based on these studies revealed that minimal or at best moderate rate of hyaline-like cartilage formation was observed once the bioactive glass implant bonded to the bone. A more promising result can be achieved through the use of porous bioactive glass implants [252].

As a result of issues such as the reactivity caused by an increase in surface area, the method of application, and chemistry associated with the bioactivity, it has been suggested that bonding can be enhanced when bioactive glass in the form of granules is used [262, 336 - 338]. Furthermore, bioactive glass granules have also been acknowledged to provide a promising alternative that can be used exclusively as a filler material to fill the gap around the implants or in bone defects [339 - 344]. On the other hand, the bone-forming capability of bioactive glass particulate according to a study by Virolainen *et al.* [342] seems to be lower compared with an autogenous bone graft.

CHAPTER 13

Surface Modifications

Abstract: Over the years, the research and applications of calcium phosphate materials as nanocoatings for dental and biomedical applications have undergone a revolution to become a state-of-the-art approach for improving osseointegration of implants and devices. Determination of stresses within a nanocoating is vital as its mechanical stability is governed by factors such as deposition method and heat treatments applied. The presence of external mechanical loading as well as the possibility of the coating to crack and spall because of inbuilt stresses (whether they are tensile or compressive) will affect the successful deployment of biomaterial implants. The most commonly used methods for characterizing the performance of micro- and nanocoatings on substrates can generally be divided into the measurement of coating properties and adhesion strength. Several excellent methods that can be used in thin film mechanical properties evaluation, and some of the commonly used methods are nanoindentation, tensile testing, scratch testing, adhesion and wear testing, pin-on-disk testing, pull-out test, and bending and bulge testing. Furthermore, the biomechanical characteristics of nanocoatings such as hydroxyapatite deposited on metallic substrates have also been examined using nanomechanical testing and nanoindentation simulated *via* the finite element approach.

Keywords: Anodization, Bone morphogenetic protein, Calcium phosphate, Collagen, Drug delivery, Finite element analysis, Hydroxyapatite HAp, Interfacial adhesion, Mechanical properties, Microtensile testing, Nanocoatings, Nanocomposite coating, Nanoindentation, Peptide, Plasma spraying, Sol-gel, Stem cell.

At the moment, dental and oral and maxillofacial implants that are currently being employed are manufactured with metallic materials such as bioinert cobalt chromium alloys or titanium alloys and do not chemically bond to bone unless modified. Consequently, they are surgically inserted and bonded with bone cements or by mechanical fixation involving micro-texturing.

The prevention of inflammatory responses is a vital requirement for dental and biomedical implants and devices regardless of the design or the implant materials used. Furthermore, an implant is also required to provide adequate biological fixation and to promote osseointegration. Surface modifications performed on

Andy H. Choi and Besim Ben-Nissan

these implant materials are intended to improve bioactivity and, if possible, protect that material against biodegradation and preventing the discharge of metal ions. Ultimately, an improved environment and structure is created which supports the regeneration of new bone [165, 216, 218, 219].

After an implantation, a number of tissue responses can occur at interfaces between the implanted biomaterial and hard or soft tissues. Various factors can influence the success rate of a dental implant or prosthesis such as the design of the implant or device, the materials used and their structure and properties, the surgical procedure or technique employed, biomechanics and application and influence of the functional loading and, last but not least, the patient's health and medical condition. Similarly, the health and well-being of the patient could be affected by the type of treatment used. The goal is to reduce the production of oxidizing species related to reactive oral diseases, which lowers the risk of oxidative-related systemic diseases [343]. A study has suggested the stress levels faced by the dental surgeon should also be considered as the quality of the performances they provide will undoubtedly be effected as well as avoiding any potential mistakes that could be made during their daily activities [344].

During the last three decades, research into surface modification to achieve rapid healing, early osseointegration, bone-implant adaptability and ultimately improving the durability and dependability of implants, is driven by concerns and issues associated with biological interactions and cell adhesions. Improvement of surfaces by increasing bioactivity with chemical and biological means and surface macro- and micro-texturing has been the major focus for many researchers in the biomedical and surgical field.

Whilst the most important factor on bone attachment is the size of micro-pores, which governs mechanical bonding and attachment, bioactivity in general can be enhanced using macro- and micro-texturing as well as calcium phosphate coatings. However, the properties and microstructure of nanostructured materials such as nanoparticles, nanocoatings and nanocomposites are governed by factors such as their synthesis or manufacturing methods, chemical composition, and structure and thickness of the coating. Surface-modified or micro-textured structures have an added advantage which involves mechanical interlocking and bonding chemically to bone under certain conditions.

13.1. NANOCOATINGS: DEFINITION

Metallic and non-metallic coatings can be classified as macro-, micro- and nanocoatings based on their thickness. Nanocoatings can be defined as thin films with a thickness between 1 to 1000 nm (1 micron), that may contain homogeneous and isotropic compounds. Scientific notation is usually mixed regarding the definitions of "thin film" coatings and "nanocoatings" and it has been quite controversial as to which term is more appropriate with no known and widely accepted explanation and both are used interchangeably [165, 216, 218, 219].

The typical thickness of a single-layered coating is less than 100 nm. Multiple-layered coatings with suitable biological, chemical, physical and mechanical properties can be simply produced. They can be applied with different compositions as nanolaminates or multilayered gradient coatings. Advantages of nanocoatings include the ease of synthesis, low cost due to the small amounts of materials needed for thin coating processes, range of deposition approaches, capacity to be integrated with different compounds and nanoparticles, and purity induced by the selection of raw ingredients [165, 216, 218, 219].

Techniques such as sol-gel, chemical vapor deposition (CVD), physical vapor deposition (PVD), metal-organic CVD, thermal or diffusion conversion, electrochemical vapor deposition, plasma and fusion coating have been applied to deposit both micro- and nanocoatings on various substrates.

Similar to orthopedic implants, all coatings deposited on dental and oral and maxillofacial implants will experience various degrees of loads and stresses applied externally. For this reason, obtaining a thorough understanding into the combined effect of the coating-substrate properties as well as the fracture resistance and strength of the coating is crucial. Undoubtedly, the substrate can be exposed to accelerated wear and corrosion due to fracture and de-adhesion of the coating, and the coating debris may trigger a negative response within human tissue. For that reason, these coatings must retain its integrity when exposed to concentrated and repeated applied loads. Obtaining an insight into the susceptibility of the coating to delamination, deformation, and fracture is vital from a clinical perspective and in the scientific community.

Depending on their intended use, different dental and biomedical devices will utilize coating materials with various functions, properties, and designs. As a result, accurate measurement methodologies are vital in determining the mechanical properties of these coatings as they can differ significantly from the bulk material. Above all, more reliable and better techniques are necessary to quantitatively determine the fracture toughness at the coating-substrate interface as well as the hardness and adhesion strength of coatings [345].

Experimental data attained from microscratch and nanoindentation tests are crucial in the characterization of coating properties at the submicron level. The knowledge gained based on these tests concerning the failure processes as well as mechanical behavior combined with other suitable characterization techniques will enable us to acquire new information on the materials used for thin films and coatings. In addition, theoretical modeling techniques such as FEA are necessary in obtaining deeper insights into the behavior at the coating-substrate interface, and this may result in better design and selection of materials used for coatings and substrates.

13.2. BIOCERAMIC COATINGS: PRODUCTION METHOD

As discussed previously, averting osteolysis and inflammatory responses in addition to promoting biological fixation and osseointegration are critical requirements for any implant, regardless whether it is ceramic, metallic, or polymeric.

Surfaces of dental implants and prostheses have undergone continuous modification. Despite the fact that dental implants and prostheses have been successfully manufactured from materials such as titanium and its ternary alloys such as Ti-6Al-4V for more than two decades, they have also been associated with aseptic inflammation in orthopedic joint replacement arguably thought to be caused by the release of titanium particles from the implant surface into the surrounding micro-environment. A recent study has shown that ultrasonic scaling of titanium implants could release particles in a surface type-dependent manner which may aggravate peri-implantitis [346]. The application of bioceramic micro- and nanoscale coatings on these materials is intended to provide protection against the release of metal ions that could trigger a negative host response.

Most importantly, their failure to adjust to the local tissue environment is a major drawback of synthetic implants, and in particular, cells do not adhere adequately or directly to most metallic surfaces. Intimate tissue ingrowth is the ideal mechanism for fixation. The purpose of utilizing calcium phosphate-based thin films and nanocoatings is to speed up the healing process by altering the surface properties of oral and dental implants and prostheses.

Surface modification and coatings on titanium are of vital importance as they permit the use of an assortment of coatings whilst conserving the favorable bulk properties of the titanium. A number of macro- and nanocoatings including sol-gel-derived ceramic coatings display promise because of their ability to provide outstanding mechanical properties attributable to their nanocrystalline structure, ability to form a chemically and physically uniform coverage over complex geometric shapes, and their relative ease of production [165, 216, 218, 219, 347].

During the past three decades, four general conventional industrial coating techniques have been projected for the manufacture of bioactive calcium phosphate coatings for clinical applications. The first technique was developed by

Ducheyne and his colleagues. The first technique was developed by Ducheyne and his colleagues. Thick calcium phosphate coatings designed for bone ingrowth were deposited using spray coating approach. The thicknesses of coatings produced are between 100 µm to 2 mm [348]. The second approach developed by Hench and his colleagues centered on the deposition of thick bioglass coatings with surface bioactivity [284].

Throughout the early 1990s, Kokubo *et al.* created the third approach that is based on self-assembly through precipitation in a simulated body fluid (SBF) solution [349]. This technique was adopted and used at a later stage to examine the biocompatibility of a range of new materials rather than as a coating. A similar method as developed by deGroot and co-workers around the same period. The forth technique developed by Ben-Nissan and co-workers for calcium phosphate nanocoatings shows very encouraging signs and is considerably newer. The method involves dipping in sol-gel-derived calcium phosphate solutions to produce strong 70 to 100 nm thick single or multi-layered nanocoatings [165, 216, 218, 219].

At the moment, coating techniques such as electrophoretic deposition, sol-gel, sputter process, dip coating, and thermal spraying have been used in the deposition of ceramic coatings. However, each offers different benefits and suffers from disadvantages that prevent it from being the ideal coating system, as shown in Table **15**.

For thick coatings, high temperature sintering of powder ceramics at 1000°C or above is necessary, which can reduce the mechanical properties of the titanium substrate. Commercially pure titanium possesses a hexagonal close-packed (HCP) crystal structure or alpha phase if the temperature is below the beta phase transus temperature or 882.5°C. Above this temperature, titanium will undergo transformation to a body-centered cubic (BCC) structure or beta phase. The subsequent strain caused by this phase transformation at that temperature will result in the degradation of the bond strength of the ceramic coating [350]. The newer sol-gel dip coating process uses much lower temperatures, and hence no transformation issues as stated above.

Currently, the primary technique used in the application of calcium phosphate coatings on medical implants is thermal or plasma spraying. This technique has had serious problems in spite of its extensive utilization. For instance, the coatings generated contain amorphous phases, highly porous, and are relatively thick. In addition, the coatings produced are usually non-uniform and have poor bonding strength to metal implants. Additionally, the dissociation of the HAp to other phases such as β-tri-calcium phosphate (TCP) and calcium oxide (CaO) has been well documented due to the fact that plasma spraying is a high temperature processing method. In comparison to HAp, these phases have a much quicker dissolution rates and will generate complications within the physiologic environment. The use of new and improved coating techniques as well as changes in the composition and the application of post-treatments have permitted plasma spraying to be successfully used to coat both dental and orthopedic implants and devices.

Table 15. Bioceramic coating techniques and thickness of coating produced.

Deposition Method	Advantages	Disadvantages	Coating Thickness
Plasma Spraying	Low cost; High deposition rate.	Line of sight technique; Amorphous coating due to rapid cooling; High temperature induces thermal decomposition.	30 - 200 µm
Sol-Gel	Complex shapes can be easily coated; No residual stresses; Homogeneous; High purity.	Post-treatment (curing) needed; Edge cracking might occur; Cannot induce mechanical interlock.	50 - 400 nm
Electrochemical Deposition	Rapid; Can coat complex shapes; Low cost; Can produce coating with uniform thickness.	The bonding between coating and substrate is not of sufficient strength.	0.05 - 0.5 mm
Sputter Deposition	Can produce a dense coating with uniform thickness on flat surface.	Process is expensive and time consuming; A line of sight technique; Low deposition rate; Generates an amorphous coating.	0.5 - 3 µm
Electrophoretic Deposition	Rapid; Can coat complex shapes; Can produce coating with uniform thickness.	Difficult to produce a crack-free coating.	0.1 - 2 mm
Pulsed Laser Deposition	Can produce both porous and dense coating; Process involves coating by crystalline and amorphous phases.	Process is expensive; A line of sight technique; Low deposition rate.	0.05 - 5 µm

13.2.1. Plasma Spraying

By far, the most widely used technique for the deposition of calcium phosphate coatings is thermal or plasma spraying. In this technique, gas plasma is generated using a variety of sources such as radiofrequency or direct current arc. The powder is heated into a partially liquid form by the plasma and it is propelled towards the substrate. Plasma spraying can be conducted in an ambient atmosphere, vacuum, or controlled atmospheres. The substrate materials can be exposed to intense heat as a result of the high temperature used during plasma spraying and this could result in residual thermal stresses in the coatings.

A number of processing routes can be applied depending on the materials used as well as on the desired performance of the coating. These processing routes include plasma spraying, high velocity oxyfuel spraying, flame spraying, and detonation flame spraying. In recent times, a more economical approach to the production of thin calcium phosphate coatings have been provided by solution and suspension thermal spraying. Compared to powder plasma sprayed coatings, suspension plasma sprayed coatings are more porous and this porosity leads to a reduction in the elastic modulus and hardness of the bulk coating. However, site specific indentations on dense areas in the suspension plasma sprayed coating carried out in a study by Gross and Saber-Samandari revealed greater values, possibly as a result of crystal orientation and finer grain size [351].

The adhesion of plasma-sprayed calcium phosphate coatings has been a primary issue for dental prostheses, cementless hip and knee. Factors determining the adhesion of thermally sprayed coatings include the distribution and size of the pores, crack population, the integrity of the coating-substrate interface, and residual stresses. A number of issues can effect the adhesion strength and several of them are related to substrate preparation, powder characteristics, and spray variables such as spray parameters [352].

During the early years, FDA placed a restriction on the manufacturing of plasma-coated calcium phosphate implants for use in dentistry owing to problems concerning the dissolution and mechanical degeneration of the splats. However, improvement in the plasma coating techniques, optimization and the use of different chemistry such as fluoro-HAp, and the application of suitable heat treatments have improved the issues concerning phase change and ultimately the dissolution.

Today, plasma spraying is used extensively on a commercial scale for the depositon of calcium phosphate coating onto dental and orthopedic implants and prostheses. Thermal spraying process produces a mixture of crystalline and amorphous phases, and this result in variable solubility determined either by the dissolving phosphate phases or by the amount of the amorphous phase.

Plasma spraying is capable of synthesizing coatings with thicknesses ranging from microns to millimeters. The thickness of commercially produced calcium phosphate coatings using thermal or plasma spraying is between 30 to 100 μm. As a result of the chemistry and thickness of the coating, adhesion and bone growth can be easily initiated. New generation nanocoatings, on the other hand, have a thickness between 70 to 200 nm. Furthermore, a permanent chemical and mechanical bonding can be created simply by depositing these coatings onto macro- and micro-textured surfaces. However, bone mechanical interlocking cannot be generated due to the thickness of the coating, but the increased surface area owing to nanostructured grains promotes faster healing and osseointegration [218, 219].

13.2.2. Sol-Gel

A versatile and attractive approach, the sol-gel method can be used to synthesize ceramic coatings such as calcium phosphate from solutions using chemical routes. Objects with complex shapes can also be coated using this method. It has also been demonstrated that both the mechanical properties and osseointegration can be enhanced as a result of the nanocrystalline grain structure produced by the sol-gel approach [218, 219].

Dating back to the beginning of chemistry, the history of the sol-gel approach (in particular for oxide coatings) begun in 1846 when it was first recognized as an application technology after Ebelmen noticed the hydrolysis and polycondensation of tetraethylorthosilicate (also referred to as tetraethoxysilane) [353]. The first patent on sol-gel describing the production of SiO_2 and TiO_2 coatings was published in 1939 [354].

In the mid-1950s, the potential of sol-gel technology was acknowledged by Roy and Roy when they discovered in their study that traditional ceramic processing techniques were not suited to produce high-purity glasses. Consequently, the notion of producing homogeneous multicomponent glasses utilizing the sol-gel approach was born [355].

13.2.2.1. The Basics

A sol can be defined as a suspension of colloidal particles within a liquid [356]. The difference between a solution and a sol is that a solution is a single-phase system, while a sol is a two-phase, solid-liquid system. The dimensions of the colloidal particles can vary between roughly 1 to 1000 nm. As a result, gravitational forces on these colloidal particles can be neglected, while surface charges and short-range forces such as van der Waals forces govern their interactions.

Stability of the system is imparted through diffusion of the colloids by Brownian motion, which leads to a low-energy arrangement [357]. The stability of the sol particles can be enhanced by reducing their surface charges. A significant reduction in the surface charge will result in gelation and the subsequent product can maintain its shape without the use of a cast.

A gel can be considered as a composite as it is composed of a solid skeleton or network that encloses a liquid phase or excess of solvent. The chemistry of gels will determine its physical and mechanical characteristics. They can be soft and possess a low elastic modulus, which can be achieved through controlling the polymerization of the hydrolyzed starting compound. The formation of a three-dimensional network will eventually lead to the creation of a high molecular weight polymeric gel. The resultant gel can be thought of as a macroscopic molecule extending throughout the solution. The gelation point can be defined as the time needed for the last bond to develop within this network. Using this gelation, a nanostructured monolith, powders, or nanosized coating can be produced based on the procedure employed (Fig. **37**) [218, 219].

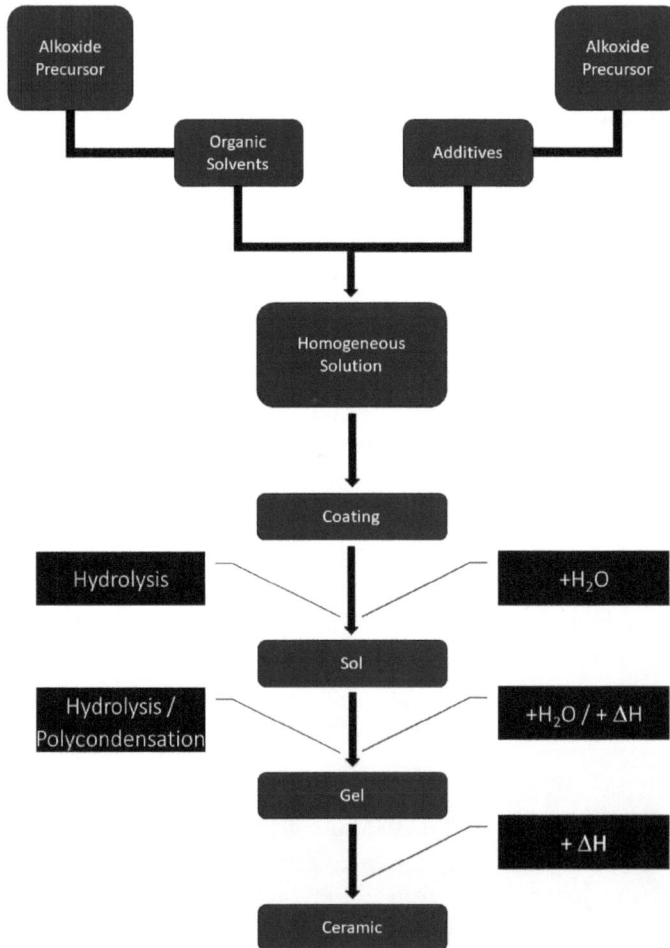

Fig. (37). The production of a thin-film ceramic coating using the sol-gel technique.

The sol-gel technique can be classified as alcohol- or aqueous-based. The presence of water is eliminated until the hydrolysis stage for the alcohol-based systems, whereas aqueous-based systems are typically performed in the presence of water. However, there are also sol-gel routes referred to as non-hydrolytics and they do not require any form of solvents.

In a similar manner, the precursors used in sol-gel can be divided into alkoxides and non-alkoxides. Precursors ideal for sol-gel productions are alkoxides because of their volatility. Furthermore, metal salts can also be utilized such as the chemical elements in Group 1 and 2 of the periodic table. In many cases, the alkoxides formed from these elements are non-volatile solids with a low solubility [357].

The synthesis of sol solutions will require the application of solvents. Normally, the solvents are organic alcohols (Fig. **37**). They are used to reduce the effect of concentration gradients, to dilute liquid precursors, and more importantly to dissolve solid precursors. Factors such as particle morphology [358] and crystallization temperatures [359] are governed by the type of solvents used.

During the synthesis of sol-gel-derived forms, a vast quantity of organic materials is required. As a result, cracking can be problematic during the production stages caused by issues such as fast drying. During drying, it is common for shrinkage to occur during the productions of monoliths. Cracking in thicker coatings however are frequently caused by issues associated with the drying process, separation of phases, as well as inhomogeneities attributable to the thermal incompatibility between the coating and substrate material.

Precursors are used to form a solution which is then used to synthesize a sol. Utilizing various deposition methods, coatings are produced from these solutions. Hydrolysis occurs once the coated substrate is exposed to water. During this stage, a three-dimensional network is created once the formation of hydroxides or hydrated oxides is complete and the gelation process ceased. Good examples are oxide coatings such as alumina and zirconia.

The process of gelation can be described as the growth of clusters through polymer condensation or particle aggregation up to a point where the clusters collide. Since no latent heat is released, an increase in viscosity is used to determine the gel point.

The next stage consists of drying and firing of the gel. Undoubtedly, drying is the most vital process in the production of monoliths using the sol-gel route. The process involves the removal of excess solvents from the pore network. During the drying and firing (sintering) of a monolith, a significant amount of shrinkage will occur, and this amount is relative to the moisture content [360].

As stated earlier, cracking can be a problem attributable to the large capillary stresses generated when pores are small, for example less than 20 nm. The vast amount of materials lost can also contribute to the cracking problem, and therefore the subsequent shrinkage that takes place [284]. This can be avoided through careful control of drying conditions, increasing the amount of cross-linking, and the use of drying control chemical additives (DCCA) (Fig. **37**).

In comparison to monoliths, it is not such an issue during the drying of sol-ge--derived nanocoatings. This is because all the shrinkage within the nanocoating will occur perpendicular to the substrate as they are constrained in the plane of the substrate [361]. Coatings with a thickness less than 400 to 500 nm can be dried at controlled rates in order to minimize the potential for cracking. However, when thickness of the films exceeds approximately 500 nm, cracking becomes difficult to avoid [362 - 365].

The critical thickness for debonding or cracking to occur in coating is defined as [366]:

$$t_{coat} = \frac{2\gamma E_{coat}}{\sigma_{coat}^2} \tag{51}$$

where t_{coat} is the thickness of the coating (or film), E_{coat} is the plain strain (elastic modulus) of the coating, γ is the fracture energy to create new surface, and σ_{coat} is the stress in the coating.

The final step in the synthesis of ceramic materials using the sol-gel route is referred to as firing or sintering. Any organic materials that remained are combusted when the dried gels are heated to an elevated temperature, typically at 600°C. Due to the small grain sizes obtained in this process, sintering temperatures are between 400°C and 800°C. Some specific chemistry allows lower temperatures such as 90°C.

13.2.2.2. Alkoxide Route

Since the early 1990s, a number of sol-gel routes have been utilized in the production of synthetic calcium phosphate coatings. As previously mentioned, the first pure calcium phosphate nanocoatings were introduced by Ben-Nissan *et al.* in 1989 and it was based on the process of Masuda *et al.* [367] on HAp powder production (Fig. **38**).

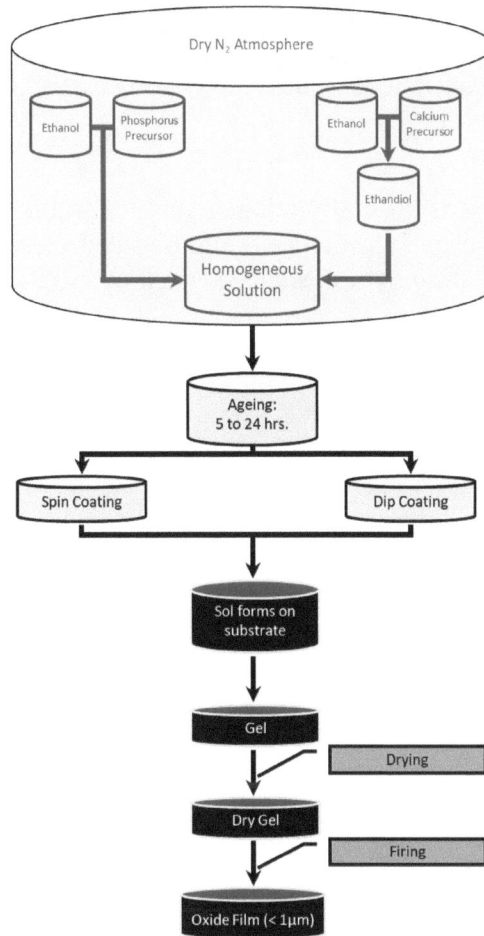

Fig. (38). The production of a calcium phosphate coating from the alkoxide route.

This method was modified in both chemistry and process to produce sound nanocoatings with highest purity and homogeneity. The precursor solution was created by mixing calcium acetate monohydrate $(Ca(OAc)_2 \cdot H_2O)$ or calcium diethoxide $(Ca(OEt)_2)$ with ethylene glycol. Once the dissolution of the calcium precursors is complete, diethyl hydrogen-phosphonate $(C_2H_5O)_2P(O)H$ is added until a stoichiometric ratio of between Ca and P of 1.67 is reached. Using the solution produced, coatings are deposited and then subjected to heat treatment at low temperatures [368, 369].

The coating technique was applied to a range of biomaterials such as 316L stainless steel, titanium alloys, cobalt chromium alloys, ceramics, glass, and a variety of calcium phosphates derived from marine structures such as coral and foraminifera for bone graft and slow drug-delivery applications [216, 218, 219].

There are two major coating techniques: dip coating and spin coating.

13.2.2.3. Dip Coating

The dip coating process is normally a batch process and is primarily used for the fabrication of coatings on items such as flat glass substrates. However, dip coating can also be used for coating complex shapes such as rods, pipes, tubes, and fibers [370].

The overall process can be broken up into five stages (Fig. **39**):

1. Immersion;
2. Start up;
3. Deposition;
4. Drainage; and
5. Evaporation

The first two steps always occur in sequence. Unless the necessary preventative measures are taken, the third and fourth steps can occur in tandem throughout the entire coating process (Fig. **39**).

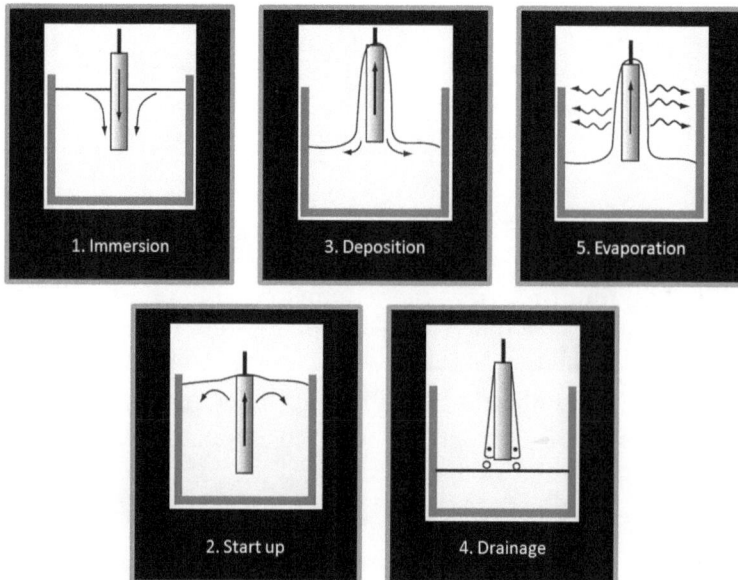

Fig. (39). Schematic showing the stages involved in a dip coating process.

The withdrawal speed will determine the thickness of a single-layered coating produced for any given solution. On the other hand, by changing the viscosity of the solution and the number of layers deposited, the thickness of the coating produced can be altered [371 - 373]. The thickness of the deposited film or coating (t_{coat}) can be determined using the following equation [370]:

$$t_{coat} = c \left(\frac{\eta U}{\rho g}\right)^{\frac{1}{2}} \tag{52}$$

where c is a constant and is about 0.8 for Newtonian liquids, η is the viscosity of the sol, U is the withdrawal speed, ρ is the density, and g is the acceleration due to gravity.

Once substrates are dip-coated, the thickness of the deposited coating will be different at the edges. This might generate cracks during firing. Faster pullout rates generate thicker coatings due to less drainage and evaporation during pullout. By proper control of the pullout rate, crack-free coatings with thicknesses between 70 to 100 nm can be produced when all other factors are adequate.

The dip coating process has the advantage of being capable of fabricating multilayered coatings with a high thickness uniformity of up to 1000 nm (Fig. **40**). In addition, multi-layered coatings can be manufactured with certain optical characteristics and are commercially utilized [364].

13.2.2.4. Spin Coating

Ideally used for flat shapes such as plates and disks, the process can be divided into four phases. The first phase involves an excess quantity of coating material delivered to the substrate surface while it is spinning or stationary. Due to the presence of centrifugal force when the substrate is spinning at maximum speed, rotation will cause the coating material to move radially outwards. The third phase involves the separation of excess material in the shape of droplets once they flow to the perimeter of the substrate. Drainage can occur if the substrate has a hole in its center similar to the dip coating process. It is worthy to mention that evaporation can occur at any given time throughout the entire deposition process.

The film or coating thins down to a fairly uniform thickness, except for the edges, which thin down due to edge effects caused by surface tension.

As the thickness of the coating decreases, the flow decreases as a result of an increase in drag forces. Evaporation can be influential to thinner coatings and becomes the key process once spinning has stopped. It will also cause the viscosity of the solution to increase by concentrating the amounts of non-volatiles present. Provided that the viscosity of the coating material is insensitive to shear rate (Newtonian behavior), a uniformity in the coating thickness will be achieved and this uniformity will take place when a balance is reached between viscous forces and centrifugal forces.

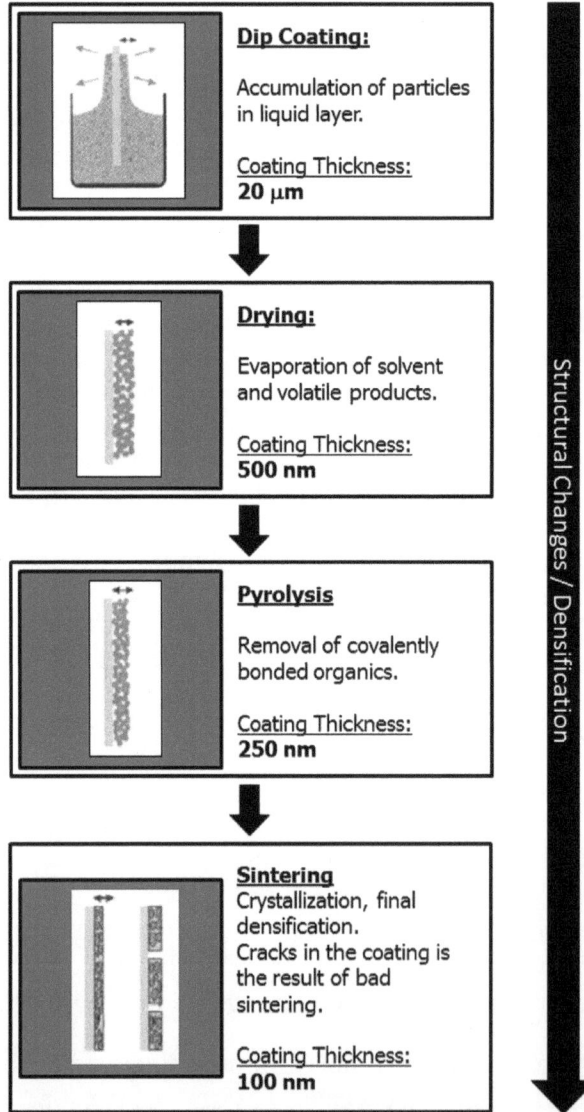

Fig. (40). Schematic showing the densification of nanocrystalline coating produced *via* the sol-gel dip coating process.

The final thickness of a spin-coated film or coating (t_{coat}) is given by [370]:

$$t_{coat} = \left(\frac{V}{V_0}\right)\left(\frac{3\eta e}{2V_0\omega}\right)^{\frac{1}{3}}$$

(53)

where V is the solvent volume fraction in the coating, V_0 is the initial solvent volume fraction, ω is the angular velocity, e is the evaporation rate, and η is the viscosity of the solution.

This equation shows that the coating thickness can be controlled by adjusting the deposition conditions (spin speed), as well as the viscosity and solids content of the solution. Under certain conditions, they can induce heterogeneities of the coatings if the metallic substrates are oxidized at different thicknesses. These areas might cause spalling or cracking of the coatings during sintering.

13.2.3. Plasma Sprayed Coating and Sol-Gel Nanocoating: Comparison

As previously mentioned, plasma spraying is without a doubt the most common technique used in the deposition of calcium phosphate micro- and macro-coatings. Plasma spraying has also been used comprehensively on a commercial scale as the primary coating process in the manufacture of dental and orthopedic implants.

Despite the fact that all of the above-mentioned problems have been resolved, one of the major concerns from a clinical perspective with plasma-sprayed calcium phosphate coatings has been centered on the adhesion of the splats generated during plasma spraying. The other concern is related to the dissociation of calcium phosphate to calcium oxide as well as other phosphate phases during the process stage. It has been well documented that these materials possess a more rapid solubility within the physiological environment. The integrity of the coating-substrate interface, distribution and size of the pores formed, residual stresses, and defect population are also important and crucial for long-term clinical stability. In addition, the strength of adhesion can be influenced by a number of different factors, such as spray parameters, substrate preparation, and powder characteristics [214, 348, 352, 374].

The adhesion or bond strength of plasma sprayed micro- and macro-coatings has been quantitatively determined using techniques such as push- and pull-off methods and micro-tensile adhesion test [345, 375].

The adhesive bond strength of plasma coatings are governed by the processing conditions and can vary from 5 to 25 MPa. Based on the findings from a number of studies, an increase in the bond strength can be achieved simply by increasing the plate power, while the bond strength decreases as the working distance increases. Using a working distance of 90 mm and a plate power of 28 kW, a maximum adhesive bond strength of 25 MPa was recorded. At the completion of a pull-off test, failures at the fracture surfaces were categorized as either adhesive (delamination at the interface between coating and substrate) or cohesive (delamination within the coating) [345].

On the contrary, it is well established that since the grain sizes at in the nanometer range, nanocrystalline coatings display superior strength, hardness, and bioactivity [216, 218, 219]. Extensive research has been conducted to determine exactly how the adhesion of sol-gel derived coatings can be increased. It has been proposed that the adhesion of calcium phosphate coatings to titanium substrates can be enhanced through the use of a TiO_2 interlayer [376 - 378].

Another key factor that has an effect on the mechanical behavior of calcium phosphate coatings is the heat treatment temperature [365]. In addition, alkali treatment is another approach that can be used to improve bonding strength and to stabilize the coating. The increase in bond strength on NaOH-treated titanium substrates has been suggested to be the result of factors such as high surface roughness as well as the formation of a thin sodium titanium oxide layer [379].

13.3. MULTI-FUNCTIONAL NANOCOMPOSITE COATINGS

As mentioned, porous bulk calcium phosphate cannot be utilized in load-bearing applications due to its unfavorable mechanical properties. Instead, calcium phosphate is used as a coating employing the ductility of the substrate metal.

Nanocomposite coating be defined as a mixture of two or more materials consisting of a matrix material and nanoscale secondary particles. It can also be produced by laminating different nanocoatings together to achieve the required coating thickness, structures, and properties. As such, one form of nanocomposite coating is a multilayered, nanolaminated mixed nanocoating.

Using the nanocomposite approach, the mechanical properties of the calcium phosphate coating can be further enhanced once other materials (micro- and/or nanoscale-based) are added to calcium phosphate as a secondary phase. In the biomedical field, the matrix must be a biocompatible biogenic, polymeric, metallic, or ceramic material.

Furthermore, it is possible using nanoparticles to manipulate the mechanical properties of the composites such as strength to match the values found in natural bone, using this composite approach. A number of fascinating possibilities in tissue engineering for oral and maxillofacial and orthopedic applications are offered by these new generation materials.

At present, this idea is being used to develop new generations of nanocomposite coatings containing natural and synthetic nanomaterials such as carbon nanotubes, bioglass, collagen, chitosan and silica to promote osseointegration and improve properties [216]. Synthetic polymers such as PLGA have also been used as secondary phases in nanocomposites with calcium phosphate. It has been suggested a nanocomposite structure consisting of calcium phosphate and polymeric material is expected to induce cellular responses at the interface with titanium implants [380]. In their investigation, they observed cells grown on surfaces coated with a nanocomposite consisting of calcium phosphate and a maleic polyelectrolyte, sodium maleate-vinyl acetate copolymer, which induced a higher proliferation rate than compared to calcium phosphate coated surfaces, indicating the improvement in surface bio-adhesion by the addition of a sodium maleate copolymer [380].

13.3.1. Applications of Biological Materials

In an effort to enhance and promote osseointegration of dental implants and the prospect of reducing the timeframe for implant integration, a greater emphasis will be placed on the incorporation of nanoscale and molecular-based biological materials such as peptides, liposomes, and bone morphogenetic proteins to calcium phosphate coatings in the future. Moreover, the additions of bone morphogenetic proteins, growth factors, stem cells and a number of pharmaceuticals are the current trends on multifunctional nanocoatings.

13.3.1.1. Stem Cells

New possibilities of producing a variety of osteoinductive hybrid "living" biomaterials is offered by combining surface coatings of amino acid functionalized calcium phosphate nanoparticles with mesenchymal stem cells (MSCs) modified directly in aqueous suspension [381]. The main challenge associated with the clinical use of MSCs is how they are obtained from healthy tissues. In recent years, the oral cavity has played a major role as an important source of MSCs. The ease of access to the dental clinicians and surgeons as well as the efficiency of cells being isolated from dental tissues such as freshly extracted teeth makes the clinical applications of oral-derived stem cells such as dental pulp stem cells extremely attractive [382]. Furthermore, a study has revealed MSCs isolated from human periapical cysts could potentially be used in bone tissue regeneration as they demonstrate the potential to differentiate into adipocyte- and osteoblast-like cells *in vitro* [383, 384]. Most importantly, a published study has suggested that both types of stems cells were able to be differentiated into odontoblast/osteoblast-like cells, confirming their vital role as new generation MSCs [385].

Viable cell/calcium phosphate conjugates in addition to plasmid DNA transfected constructs can be produced simply and efficiently using a three-dimensional coating strategy method [381]. Their study indicated that MSC differentiation and bone matrix production in the absence of osteogenic media is sufficiently stimulated by the bioinorganic coating. In comparison to two-dimensional approach involving adherent cells, an enhancement in gene expressions is possible by combining coated cell aggregates with specific biomolecular stimuli. Moreover, they suggested this approach can be applied to primary human cells and a new generation of biomaterials for bone tissue engineering can be created using the resultant hybrid microparticles as starting points.

13.3.1.2. Collagen

It has been hypothesized that a composite coating composed of collagen and calcium phosphate could be beneficial by imitating the unique nanocomposite structure of human bone tissue. Furthermore, the poor fracture toughness of calcium phosphate could be counterbalanced by the ductile properties of collagen [306, 386, 387].

In a study, nanometer-thick calcium phosphate and collagen-calcium phosphate composite coatings were deposited on titanium substrates using a collagen/calcium phosphate ratio comparable to that of native bone tissue [388]. It was discovered the co-deposition of collagen could significantly improve the adhesive and cohesive strength of calcium phosphate coatings. Similar to calcium phosphate coatings, their study also revealed collagen-calcium phosphate composite coatings could stimulate osteogenic behavior *in vitro* upon cell culture testing using rat bone marrow cells even when the thickness of the coating was below 100 nm. In addition, an improvement in osteoblast differentiation was also achieved based on a decrease in proliferation and accelerated mineral deposition when compared to pure calcium phosphate coatings.

In another study, the bone formation around a calcium phosphate-collagen nanocomposite coated titanium rod placed under the periosteum of a rat calvarium was studied [389]. The result of a bonding strength test revealed the calcium phosphate-collagen coated specimens generated the highest bonding strength to bone than uncoated and calcium phosphate coated specimens. Furthermore, the collagen-calcium phosphate coated specimens were practically surrounded by new bone tissue without encapsulation and had the highest ratio of bone contact four weeks after surgery, while the uncoated titanium and calcium phosphate-coated specimens were encapsulated with fibrous tissues.

13.3.1.3. Bone Morphogenetic Proteins

Bone morphogenetic proteins (BMPs) are multi-functional growth factors and their roles in cellular functions in postnatal and adult animals have been comprehensively investigated in recent years. BMPs belong to the superfamily of transforming growth factor β (TGFβ) [302, 390]. In 1965, the activities of BMPs were first discovered by Urist [391], but it was not after the cloning of human BMP-2 and BMP-4 and the purification and sequencing of bovine BMP-3 (osteogenin) during the late 1980s that the proteins accountable for bone induction were recognized [392 - 394].

Originally isolated from demineralized bone matrix, recombinant human bone morphogenetic protein-2 (rhBMP-2) is capable of stimulating cell differentiation into osteoblasts and chrondroblasts in order to initiate bone and cartilage formation [394 - 396]. The recombinant human bone morphogenetic protein can be considered as one of the most investigated proteins on the preclinical and clinical scale for dental and oral and maxillofacial applications such as mandibular reconstruction and maxillary sinus floor augmentation [397 - 401]. The possibility of predicting dental implant osseointegration has been lifted by the introduction of rhBMP technology [402 - 405].

A poor surface reactivity and a very low specific surface area is displayed by commercial calcium phosphate ceramics when sintered at a high temperature. Their osteoinductive properties appear rather weak even though they are exceptional osteoconductive materials. In a groundbreaking work by Rey *et al.* [406], they hypothesized the surface and biological properties of these ceramics can be enhanced through the deposition of a nanocrystalline carbonated apatite coating. Results from physico-chemical analyses revealed such a coating could encourage biological activity by stimulating the formation of nanopores and increasing the specific surface area. Improvements in surface reactivity was confirmed in an adsorption study using an osteogenic growth factor, rhBMP-2. The amount of protein adsorbed increased and its release was sustained. *In vitro* study validated the biocompatibility of the coated ceramics. Using an ovine animal model, the *in vivo* osteoinductive property of the modified ceramic was examined in intramuscular sites. Bone formation was enhanced using the modified ceramics combined with BMP-2.

A number of clinicians and researchers proposed the possibility of utilizing a biomimetic calcium phosphate coating to transport growth factors such as BMP in an attempt to improve peri-implant bone regeneration. It has been revealed that BMP is able to incorporate and slowly releasing signaling factors during *in vivo* degradation [407, 408]. A well-established ectopic (subcutaneous) ossification model in rats was utilized to investigate the *in vivo* osteoinductive capability of a biomimetic coating containing BMP-2. Their findings revealed BMP-2 is able to be discharged from the coating *in vivo* at a steady pace and at a quantity which is sufficient to induce bone formation at an ectopic site. More importantly, the coating is capable of performing this task with a high degree of efficacy and at a low pharmacological level. It is also able to sustain this osteogenic activity for an extended period [407]. On the contrary, utilizing calcium phosphate coating to deliver BMP-2 has no substantial influence on the osteoconductivity of implants during the early phase of osseointegration as results of their later study revealed [408]. After 3 weeks of implantation, the volume of bone deposited within the peri-implant space and the bone-interface coverage was greatest for implants coated with calcium phosphate containing no BMP-2. Titanium implants with no coatings and implants with BMP-2 adsorbed onto the calcium phosphate coating produced the least amount of bone-interface coverage and bone deposited.

A much greater osteogenic surface environment on titanium surfaces can be generated using the combined efforts of osteoinductive BMP-2 and osteoconductive apatite as previous suggested [409]. In an effort to maintain the release rate of growth factors, a BMP-2 nanocomplex nanoparticle is formed by coupling BMP-2 with negatively charged chondroitin sulfate. Compared to calcium phosphate-coated titanium and titanium surfaces alone, cell proliferation was quicker once mouse osteoblast cells were seeded on surfaces coated with calcium phosphate containing BMP-2 nanocomplex. The use of BMP-2 nanocomplex also upregulated gene expressions of bone-specific markers (osteocalcin and type I collagen) significantly. Similar observation was also made during the assessment of alkaline phosphatase activity.

In addition to biomimetic coatings, calcium phosphate coatings produced using conventional techniques combined with rhBMP-2 have also been assessed for their possible enhancement in osseointegration of implants. Calcium phosphate coating deposited using plasma spraying combined with rhBMP-2 was postulated to result in a significant improvement in bone apposition if the implant is immersed into a protein solution prior to implantation [410]. After 3 weeks of implantation, *in vivo* observations confirmed coatings containing rhBMP-2 produced the highest bone-to-implant contact and bone area fraction occupancy. On the other hand, bone response was not significantly enhanced when rhBMP-2 was directly adsorbed onto the surfaces of titanium implants; however, it is remarkably greater than uncoated implants.

It has been previously shown that the use of combined angiogenic such as vascular endothelial growth factor (VERF) and osteogenic factor delivery promoted greater bone formation [411]. This hypothesis was later examined in a study by Ramazannoglu *et al*. where a combination of recombinant human VERF (rhVEGF) and rhBMP-2 was delivered using an implant coated with a biomimetically-derived octacalcium phosphate [412]. The combined delivery of rhBMP-2 and rhVEGF significantly improved the bone volume density around the implant in the final observation period. However, when the results of the bone-implant contact rates were compared, such a positive effect was not recorded.

13.3.1.4. Peptides

Biomimetic peptides such as RGD and P-15 have also been utilized in addition to proteins as an alternative approach to bio-functionalize implant surfaces to achieve improvements in the interactions between cells and biomaterial. Only a cell-binding sequence is contained within these biomimetic active peptides. They can be purified with relative ease and can be manufactured synthetically [413 - 416].

By biologically mimicking cell-binding sites, the RGD (Arg-Gly-Asp) peptide has been suggested to promote cell adhesion [417]. It has been previously suggested that the attachment and differentiation of osteoblasts on implant surfaces can be enhanced through the deposition of calcium phosphate coating along with an RGD containing peptide [414]. The presence of peptide was found to reinforce the osseoconductivity of calcium phosphate. The protein absorption on calcium phosphate surfaces once implanted in bone is changed after the peptide pretreatment. An increase in osseointegration may be the result of cells such as osteoprogenitors attaching preferentially to the surfaces of calcium phosphate.

In spite of *in vitro* studies suggesting improvements in cell attachment using RGD, the findings from a study by Schliephake *et al*. [418] showed there is only weak evidence suggesting peri-implant bone formation in the alveolar process could be enhanced once titanium implants are coated with RGD peptides. A similar observation was noticed in the *in vivo* study by Elmengaard *et al*. [419]. Despite the fact that a significant bone stimulating effect can be produced by cyclic RGD at the bone-implant interface, an increase in bone density was not detected outside the interface. Later, a question was raised by Hennessy *et al*. regarding the potential benefits associated with functionalizing calcium phosphate with RGD peptides on osseointegration of implants [420]. Total bone formation was restrained in a significant manner when calcium phosphate disks containing RGD was implant into rat tibiae. The amount of new bone directly contacting the implant perimeter was also constrained.

Petrie *et al*. [421] hypothesized that unregulated or sub-optimal integrin binding resulted in uncontrolled signaling responses at the tissue-implant interface. This in turn created these marginal healing responses. Moreover, Dettin *et al.* [422] also suggested peptides adsorbed onto titanium failed to promote osteoblast adhesion might be the result of structural changes in peptides as a response to surface characteristics or low peptide adsorption.

Consequently, an alternative peptide sequence, the 15-residue peptide derived from a triple helical region, 766GTPGPQGIAGQRGVV780, of the collagen α1(I) chain, is of great interest and shows great promise for implant coating applications. In the challenge against collagen for cell binding, the P-15 sequence was found to be more potent than RGD-containing peptides [415, 416, 423]. An investigation was carried out to establish the fact that coating the surfaces of dental implants with calcium phosphate and P-15 peptide will lead to a speedier osseointegration process. Histomorphometric analysis revealed that a noticeably higher percentage of bone-to-implant contact was observed on implants with high concentration of P-15 after 14 and 30 days of implantation into the forehead region of 12 adult pigs. At 30 days, an increase in peri-implant bone density was observed on implants containing both low and high concentrations of P-15 peptide [415]. These observations were later confirmed in another study that utilized a canine model to examine the influence of P-15 added to the surface of an electrochemically deposited calcium phosphate coating. Higher bone-to-implant contact was observed after one week of implantation, confirming the hypothesis that the bioactivity of a calcium phosphate-coated implant can be improved using P-15 and the effects were noticeable particularly during the early stages of the healing period [416].

13.3.2. Drug Delivery

In the past, the classical approach regarding systemic drug delivery has created a number of issues such as the influence of the dissolving drugs to the whole system rather than pinpoint local delivery. Consequently, these problems can be resolved through the application of local or targeted drug delivery. Targeting is usually achieved with appropriate functionalizing of the surfaces. Moreover, targeting these drugs directly to the required locations has the possibility of improving drug efficacy and efficiency locally aside from reducing the harm of toxicity on healthy cells within the whole environment, resulting in significant cost savings for the healthcare system.

The rapid dissolution of the carrier system within the human body sometimes limits the efficiency and the targeting capability of any drug delivery system. The main concern for drug carriers (both local and systemic delivery) is the long circulation time within the blood. As a result, a number of studies were carried out to investigate different approaches that can be utilized during the design and synthesis of the so-called "long circulating time" carriers. Amongst these approaches, the most effective way to sustain the life of drug delivery particles for prolonged periods in the blood is to modify the surfaces of carriers using thin films or nanocoatings based on non-ionic surfactant or polymeric macromolecules [424]. Nevertheless, appropriate and effective modifications of nanoparticles using multifunctional thin films and nanocoatings are essential for drug delivery systems and devices in the future.

Modification of the critical pore size and interconnectivity of a bioceramic can improve the delivery and dispersion of a material such as drugs to the targeted area. Depending on the intended areas to be targeted and delivered such as long bones and the pharmaceuticals used, these pores may range from a few nanometers to micron sizes.

As discussed earlier, due to the chemical similarity between calcium phosphate and human hard tissues, delivery systems based on such materials would permit an increase in drug efficacy while reducing toxicity to non-diseased cells at the same time. As a result of their high surface areas, nano drug-delivery systems irrespective of whether a matrix is embedded or not is able to deliver and regulate its dissolution with a high degree of precision [425, 426].

Controlling the rates of dissolution as well as identifying a suitable rate within the human body is the primary issue for drug carriers containing nanoparticles and nanocoatings [427]. Utilizing calcium phosphate as a delivery vehicle also expands its proficiency due to its ability to deliver minerals locally as well as other active ions such as magnesium and strontium, not to mention calcium and phosphate. If required, they can also be used to deliver biogenic materials such as stem cells and bone morphogenetic proteins in the successful treatment of bone diseases. Furthermore, calcium phosphate-based drug delivery system has an added advantage in the repair and regeneration of bone tissue, and as discussed in the previous chapter, the most appropriate bone substitutes are based on calcium phosphate materials [308, 425, 426]. They offer ease of production, able to carry drugs, and a source of both calcium and phosphates during dissolution. More importantly, they can be added to nanocoatings and thin films [428, 429].

For applications in slow drug delivery in general, a number of biological, physical, and/or chemical surface modification techniques can be employed to modify and functionalize the surfaces of nanocoatings and nanostructured materials. In addition, novel material functions and properties can be discovered through surface modifications. The stability and long-term solubility of nanocoatings in aqueous medium can also be regulated and improved *via* this approach.

It has been widely accepted in the medical and dental communities that wound contamination and postoperative infections during fracture repair or after implantation as issues that could lead to serious clinical problems and could endanger the osseointegration of implants and prostheses. As a result, antibiotics are often used as prophylactics administered either orally or intravenously.

Undoubtedly, the complication commonly and frequently associated with the application of implantable medical devices in dentistry and oral and maxillofacial surgery is bacterial infection. It has been well documented that *Pseudomonas aeruginosa* (*P. aeruginosa*) is believed to cause infections related to indwelling device particularly catheters due to the fact that it is an opportunistic pathogen. Complications arising from serious infections such as severe deep-seated infections (endocarditis, osteomyelitis and other metastatic infections), severe sepsis, and septic-thrombosis on the other hand are believed to the result of *Staphylococcus aureus* (*S. aureus*) infection.

During basic surgical and hospital treatments, one of the basic biofilm infections that can be acquired are those related to *S. aureus* and *Staphylococcus epidermidis* (*S. epidermidis*) strains, and these include *methicillin-resistant S. aureus* (MRSA). A comprehensive and thorough understanding of the molecular foundations of biofilm formation as well as their adhesion to implants will assist us in the fight against biofilm infections.

The creation of a bacterial biofilm is the source behind the development of bone infection. Within this biofilm, bacteria can differentiate into sessile forms from planktonic. As soon as the antibiotic treatment has stopped, bacteria in this sessile form can protect certain bacterial cells from releasing out of the biofilm. Bacteria adhesion is a complex phenomenon that can be influenced by a number of factors including the surface properties of materials, characteristics of the bacteria themselves, and the environmental conditions where the adhesion takes place such as in the presence of serum protein or bactericidal substance [430].

Several proposed model and theory of bacterial adhesion appear to be restricted as they disregard the biological perspectives of adhesion and only consider the physical interactions amongst the bacteria and surface. Adhesins are the specific bacterial structures that are responsible for adhesive activities as well as controlling cell to abiotic or cell-to-cell surface adhesion. For different surfaces, bacteria may have different adhesives or different acceptors. The charge of the substrate and the cell wall is determined by the ionic strength and pH of the media where the adhesion is occurring, which is governed by factors such as surface chemistry, hydrophobicity, and charge, and consequently influences their interaction.

In order to mitigate biofilm infections, various techniques on either controlling and/or preventing bacterial infections have been suggested. Methods based on the synthesis of thin films or nanocoatings with surface properties that act against microbial adhesion or viability show promise in the prevention of device-related infections. Modifying surfaces of medical implants and devices to render them resistant to microbial adhesion was another approach that has been proposed, and this modification can be achieved *via* chemical, biological, or physical means.

From a clinical perspective, the perfect coating on implants should provide several key improvements to the surgeons, such as providing a suitable antimicrobial characteristic and at the same time support actions which prevent the formation of biofilms as well as the development of post-operative infections. It is also beneficial if the coating can provide anchorage during the initial stages with suitable bioactivity including osteoconduction and osteoinduction where possible. Consequently, the utilization of multifunctional thin films or nanocoatings would be ideal in this regard.

The search has been continuous for a system capable of delivering antibiotics safely and efficiently without affecting the entire body and issues associated with long-term intravenous (IV) access. The most precise way to examine the effectiveness of an antibiotic against a disease, for example bone infections such as osteomyelitis, is to use test methods that considers evidence supporting the formation of new bone tissues during histological examination, and a prerequisite for success is the complete destruction of the infection.

Due to their capacity to degrade over time and the ability for minerals and pharmaceuticals to be absorbed and released, the use of bioceramic-biodegradable polymer thin films has been proven beneficial in the battle against biofilm infection. More importantly, the rates of drug release could be tailored to suit individual treatment plans simply by fine-tuning the sizes and interconnectivity of pores within these bioceramic particles. These bioceramic-biodegradable polymer thin film composites would be an ideal candidate in drug delivery for the repair of bone because of the bioactive nature of the bioceramic which can also accelerate the osseointegration process and the minerals added (for example magnesium, zinc, and strontium) which promote tissue growth. Recently, in an effort to prevent implant-related infections, biodegradable polymer thin films loaded with antibiotics such as gentamicin have been investigated to serve as a "composite coating" for metallic implants and fracture fixation devices [429, 431 - 433].

However, the inadequate diffusion and penetration of antibiotics across the biofilm is believed to be the reason behind the perseverance of biofilm infections, and in particular, infections related to implantable devices [434, 435]. A number of reasons have been postulated regarding the microbial resistance to antimicrobial agents. A number of reasons have been postulated regarding the microbial resistance to antimicrobial agents. A multi-layered defense based on the creation of persister cells, reducing the amounts of oxygen and nutrients available causing the bacterial to grow slowly, and adaptive stress responses has been theorized. At the moment, neutralizing biofilm resistance is the primary objective researchers are focusing on, this in turn will enhance the capabilities of antibiotics that are currently used in the treatment of biofilm-related infections [436]. In most cases, chronic suppressive therapy can be used to treat biofilm. The use of antibiotics has been reported to be effective in the prevention of biofilm during the initial stages. In order to make biofilms more susceptible to treatments, a study by Mah *et al.* [437] has suggested the appropriate manner will be to use drugs which inhibit biofilm-specific resistance together with traditional antibiotics.

13.4. MECHANICAL EXAMINATIONS OF MICRO- AND NANOCOATINGS

The magnitude of adhesive forces that occur during deposition of coating to the substrate and during the subsequent drying and firing process is determined by the nature of the coating used as well as the surfaces of the substrate. Overall, these forces can be categorized as either primary interatomic bonds such as ionic and covalent bonds or secondary bonds such as van der Waals bonding [438 - 440].

In comparison to secondary bonds, a much higher adhesion is offered by primary interatomic bonds. This is due to the fact that secondary bonds are based on much weaker physical forces categorized by dispersion forces or hydrogen bonds. Interfacial dispersion forces are produced by all surfaces, whereas hydrogen bonds normally occur on polar material surfaces.

The force holding the coating and substrate together (or any two objects) might be the result of mechanical interlocking, chemical bonding through diffusion, or electrostatic attraction. Depending on the chemistry and physical condition of both the coating used and the surface of the substrate, a combination of one or more of these proposed mechanisms may be involved [439].

Once an intimate contact is achieved between two different materials, the two free surfaces are sacrificed to create a new interface. The bond strength produced is related to the nature of interactions observed at the interface between the two materials. During any coating deposition process, a range of reactions can take place on the surface of the coating. Moreover, the adhesion and bonding between the coating and substrate can be influenced by a number of factors such as surface interactions and topography, and wettability. The ability for one phase to wet another will considerably regulate the level of these interactions. Wetting is a condition essential for adhesion.

Thermodynamic conditions can be used to define the wetting of a surface. Vital variables such as the surface tension of the coating while it is in the liquid state and the energetics of the surfaces of both the substrate and solid coating will influence the development of interfacial bonding and adhesion [439, 441]. The capacity for a liquid to spread and wet a solid is determined by the spreading coefficient. Given the fact that a relationship exists between the spreading coefficient and the surface tension, it is important to determine the surface tension of both substances as it will govern if the liquid is able to wet the solid surface or not.

The ability for a liquid coating to wet a solid surface completely is governed by the contact angle. If a greater molecular attraction occurs between liquid and solid molecules than between similar liquid molecules, then complete wetting will occur. In this case, the contact angle is zero and the liquid is able to spread over a surface without any restrictions.

The viscosity of a liquid phase is also extremely important especially in cases where the coating is in the liquid state during deposition. Consequently, wetting can be thought of as an intimate relationship between the coating and substrate. To achieve an adequate adhesion between the coating and substrate, it is vital that intimate bonding and wetting remain intact after the deposition of coating in addition to initial wetting. The mechanisms of adhesion can only become operational when there is a presence of effective wetting between the coating and the substrate.

13.4.1. Interfacial Adhesion of a Coating-Substrate System

In the context of this chapter, the mechanical bond strength between a coating (both micro- and nanocoating) and a substrate will be used as the definition of adhesion. In order to separate the coating and the substrate, a force must be applied and used to drive a crack propagating at the coating-substrate interface. This driving force can be from externally applied stresses or through internal residual stresses.

Interfacial adhesion between the coating and substrate has a vitally important role to play on the performance and reliability of medical and dental devices and products. The work of adhesion (ω_a) can be used to define the energy needed to fracture the interface between a coating and a substrate. It can be determined using the surface energies of the coating (γ_{coat}), substrate (γ_{sub}), and at the interface (γ_{inter}):

$$\omega_a = \gamma_{coat} + \gamma_{sub} - \gamma_{inter} \tag{54}$$

This is identical to the "Griffith fracture" in which the work of adhesion is the same as the fracture resistance of the interface [442]. In contrast, factors such as plastic deformation, surface roughness, asperity contacts, and bridging ligaments are not taken into consideration in the work of adhesion despite the fact that they are extremely important [443].

As a result, the practical work of adhesion (ω_p) is a more valid determination of adhesion. The practical work of adhesion is also referred to as the strain energy release rate or interfacial toughness. It can be calculated using the energy spent in plastically deforming the substrate (Ω_{sub}) and the coating (Ω_{coat}):

$$\omega_p = \omega_a + \Omega_{sub} + \Omega_{coat} \tag{55}$$

13.4.2. Adhesion Based on Mechanical Theory

A coating is believed to possess mechanical interlocking or keying characteristics when it penetrates the surfaces of the substrate material comprising of pores, scratches, crevices, and voids. This mechanism of coating adhesion is dependent on the roughness of the surface of the substrate material. Several surface analytical techniques have shown that the coating can undoubtedly penetrate into complex tunnel-shaped cracks and undercut which provides mechanical attachment upon setting and/or firing [439].

As discussed above, surface roughness will have an effect on the area available at the coating-substrate interface as well as the force a substrate is able to generate to grip the coating within the actual contact area at the interface. For that reason, the adhesion of a coating can be increased by enlarging the surface area. If the coating is able to penetrate completely into all the crevices produced during surface roughening, then the process is considered advantageous. On the other hand, voids can be generated at the interface between the coating and substrate if the coating fails to fully penetrate into the crevices. This will lead to the creation of a non-uniform coating, which has a smaller coating-to-interface contact than the actual geometric area.

13.4.2.1. Nanocoating and Surface Topography

It was demonstrated that the deposition of nanocoatings over meso- and nano-porous structures enhances the performance and mechanical properties as a consequence of pore-filling effect of the nanocoatings. More importantly, a reduction in surface defects can be achieved by covering the structure with nanocoatings and an improvement in properties of ceramic materials can also be accomplished as the nanocoatings penetrate into the meso- and nano-pores.

In the same way, the applications of nanocoatings on metallic substrates such as titanium implants can have a number of advantages over polycrystalline large grain coated materials. Nanocoated materials have large surface areas as a result of their extremely low grain size, and this in turn lowers their densification or sinter temperatures. For this reason, they can be sintered at a lower cost and at lower temperatures.

In addition, surface morphologies and small crystalline grain structures of nanocoated materials can have an effect on the biological properties as they can accelerate the bonding of the implant to hard and soft tissues as well as promoting early osseointegration in clinical applications.

Above all, the deposition of a ceramic oxide nanocoating can alter the electrical or thermal insulating properties that are advantageous in many dental and biomedical applications. For instance, the presence of a non-conductive oxide coating on dental implant can stop or reduce the metal ion release, which is a serious concern in clinical applications.

13.4.2.2. Anodizing Process

According to its electrochemical characteristics and where it is situated with the periodic table, titanium is categorized as an oxide film former [444]. In simple terms, titanium is a metal whose surface is always covered by an oxide layer formed naturally once it is exposed to an environment that contains oxygen such as water and air. The composition of the metal and manufacturing conditions used during the working of the metal such as the atmosphere and maximum temperature reached will govern the thickness of this "natural" oxide film on titanium and can vary between 5 and 70 nm [445, 446].

As a biomaterial in general, titanium relies upon the formation of an oxide layer which in principle is titanium oxide or TiO_2. More importantly, the addition of trace or alloying elements during titanium metal production can either interfere or enhance this hard adherent TiO_2 layer. This in turn determines whether the biocompatibility and corrosion resistance for a particular titanium alloy will be enhanced or reduced in comparison to commercially pure titanium metal [447, 448].

Titanium alloys are commonly used for dental and biomedical applications and a range of surface modification techniques from mechanical to chemical are commonly used. Anodizing is a method of converting the titanium alloy metal surfaces to an oxide layer to accelerate the bonding of the additional coatings including nanocoatings.

Anodic oxidation, or more commonly known as anodizing, is a well-established technique used to produce a variety of protective oxide layers on metals. It can be employed to produce thick oxide layers as porous coatings, as well as reducing the release of metal ions and to protect the metal against corrosion. The combined efforts of an electrical field and electrode reactions forces the oxygen and metal ions to diffuse, this in turn produces an oxide film on the surface of the anode [449].

The anodic oxidation of titanium are governed by rules and regulations which are very similar to the ones used for other "value" metals and the first step involves the formation on the metal surface an adsorbed layer of oxygen or some oxygenated species. It should be stated more accurately that the oxidized layer is formed on top of a pre-existing "natural" oxide layer [450, 451]. During the anodization of titanium, the chemical reactions that can take place are shown in Table **16**.

Table **16**. The main reactions leading to oxidation at the anode can be represented as follows [449].

Reaction	Equation
At Ti/Ti oxide interface:	$Ti \Leftrightarrow Ti^{2+} + 2e^-$
At Ti oxide/electrolyte interface:	$2H_2O \Leftrightarrow O^{2-} + 4H^+$ (Oxygen ions react with Ti to form oxide) $2H_2O \Leftrightarrow O_2(g) + 4H^+ + 4e^-$ (Oxygen gas evolves at the surface)
At both interface:	$Ti^{2+} + 2O^{2-} \Leftrightarrow TiO_2 + 2e^-$

The chemical and structural properties of anodic oxides on titanium can vary significantly based on the processing parameters such as the anode potential, temperature, current, and electrolyte composition. Diluted acids of H_2SO_4, H_3PO_4, and acetic acid are some of the examples of the widely used electrolytes for anodic oxidation of titanium [449].

Using an electric field applied externally, the ions of titanium and oxide generated during these redox reactions are forced through the oxide layer. This results in the growth of the oxide film. Compared to the metallic elements of the electrical circuit and the electrolyte, a noticeable reduction in the applied voltage will be observed across the oxide film at the anode as a result of the high resistivity characteristic of the anodic titanium oxides.

The current will flow and the film will grow continuously if that electric field is powerful enough to force the ions across the oxide [449]. This is the rationale behind the existence of an almost linear relationship between the applied voltage (V_{appl}) and the thickness of the final oxide film (t_{oxide}):

$$t_{oxide} = \alpha V_{appl} \tag{56}$$

where α is a growth constant, typically between 1.5 to 3.0 nm V^{-1}.

If the applied voltage is approximately 100 to 150 V, which is below the dielectric breakdown limit of the oxide, then this linear relationship is valid subjected to the electrolyte used and the processing environment [449, 452]. The oxide will not be sufficiently resistive to avoid further oxide growth and current flow if the voltage used during the anodization process is above the breakdown limit. Frequent sparking and an increase in gas evolution will result if the process is carried out at such high voltages. Typically, this form of anodization is known as spark anodizing. In comparison to anodizing conducted at voltages below the dielectric breakdown limit, spark anodizing will produce oxide films which are more porous and less uniform [449].

In addition, an equation has also been derived that describes the relationship between the anodic current across the oxide film at low anodic potentials and the electric field [453, 454]:

$$i_c = E \cdot A \exp B \tag{57}$$

where i_c is the ionic current, E is the field strength, and A and B are constants.

There is evidence supporting the notion that the anodic film on titanium grows because of Ti^{2+} cations being transferred through the film, which means that the growth takes place at the oxide surface interface [455, 457]. On the other hand, this fact has been disputed and it was believed that the growth of the film is due to oxide ion transfer [458, 459]. Furthermore, it has also been suggested that the likelihood of the ion transfer of both Ti^{2+} and O^{2-} contributing simultaneously to the growth mechanism, which is similar to that of oxidation in a gas [444].

The role electrolyte plays in the formation of the anodic film has not been investigated in great details. Both the initial passivation and the subsequent growth stages are influenced by the nature of the anions [460 - 462].

The formation of an anodic layer has also been suggested as long as the circumstances, for instance the characteristics of the electrolyte, support the creation of Ti^{4+} in the final oxide film produced instead of Ti^{3+} ions and Ti^{2+} ions [463].

13.4.3. Other Adhesion Theories

Depending on the material properties and curing conditions, atoms will diffuse to a certain extent across the interface once molecular contact through wetting is achieved between the coating and substrate. This phenomenon is a two-stage process, involving wetting followed by the creation of a chemical bond as a consequence of elements inter-diffusing across the interface [439, 441].

The formation of an electrostatic force is possible in the form of an electrical double layer at the coating-substrate interface. Residual electric charges are retained within the surfaces of both the coating and substrate which are scattered all over the system. The interactions amongst these electric charges could explain for certain adhesion of coatings [439, 441].

It is anticipated that chemical bonding is the toughest and the most durable and quite often it is possible for covalent bonds to form across the interface between substrate and coating. On the other hand, the existence of mutually reactive chemical groups firmly bounded to the surfaces of coatings and substrates are required for chemical bonding. Interfacial shims or additives can accelerate the process. It is also possible for certain surface containing various chemical functional groups (for example, some plastics, composites, and previously coated surfaces) to form chemical bonds with the substrate material during suitable conditions [441].

13.4.4. Stresses in Coatings

The determinations of stresses in coatings are of vital importance with respect to mechanical stability as a consequence of the deposition process and the temperatures involved. The stresses developed in a coating consist of three parts [464]:

1. Intrinsic: it is the consequence of issues such as deposition, structure, and mode of growth;
2. Thermal stress: the discrepancy in thermal expansion between the coating and substrate; and
3. Stresses which are applied externally.

Once the values of intrinsic stress (σ_i), thermal stress (σ_t), and any externally applied stress (σ_e) are determined, the stress generated within a coating (σ_{coat}) can be calculated using:

$$\sigma_{coat} = \sigma_i + \sigma_t + \sigma_e \qquad (58)$$

Stress measurement by substrate curvature is a simple technique that requires a phase shifting interferometer or a stylus profilometer capable of scans 10 mm in length or more. The use of optical methods such as interferometry is advantageous as it is a straightforward approach to use and offers high accuracy of about six nm and substrates with curvature of up to three μm are acceptable.

A relatively thin substrate is needed when using stylus profilometry to measure the curvature adequately. This technique requires precise and careful placement of the sample to facilitate for a cross-scan in the x- and y-directions, preferably on both sides, before and after the deposition of the coating.

A formula was suggested that could be used to describe the relationship between the changes in the curvature radius of an uncoated as well as a coated substrate and the resultant stress in the later [465]. The combined intrinsic and thermal stresses in the coating can be evaluated without any prior knowledge of the coating properties using this equation except for information such as the elastic modulus (E_{sub}) and Poisson's ratio (v_{sub}) of the substrate, the thickness of both the coating (t_{coat}) and substrate (t_{sub}), and the radius of curvature before (R_b) and after coating (R_a):

$$\sigma = \frac{1}{6}\left[\frac{1}{R_a} - \frac{1}{R_b}\right]\frac{E_{sub}}{(1 - v_{sub})}\frac{t_{sub}^2}{t_{coat}} \tag{59}$$

Using the following equation (eq. (60)), the radius (R) can be calculated assuming that the length of the substrate (L_{sub}) is much greater than the final bow (B):

$$R = \frac{L_{sub}^2}{8B} \tag{60}$$

Tensile stress in the coatings results in concave deflection, and vice versa, compressive stress leads to a convex deflection. Through the use of the deflection approach, measurements can be obtained *in situ* during deposition of the coating or subsequent thermal treatment by means of interferometry or a cantilever beam and a low-power laser. Similarly, elastic strain in the coating can be determined using X-ray diffraction from variations in crystal lattice *d*-spacing, and the information obtained such as strain-free lattice spacing and the elastic modulus can then be used to calculate the stress in the coating. On the other hand, those values may not be known in some cases [466].

13.4.5. Adhesion and Mechanical Testing Techniques

Dependable and vigorous procedures are needed to mechanically characterize coatings and nanocoatings as the demand imposed by their use in dentistry and oral and maxillofacial surgery continues to grow. With the increasing trend towards the deposition of thin films and nanocoatings on tinier devices, significant developments in the methodologies and equipment have been made. This advancement has permitted the extraction of mechanical and adhesive behaviors of coatings.

Gaining an in-depth understanding of the long-term mechanical reliability of biomedical micro- and nanocoatings is vital in clinical applications. Consequently, various techniques are required to measure quantitatively the mechanical and adhesion properties of coatings. Since the 1980s, there have been continuous developments and enhancements in the equipment capable of extracting the properties and adhesion of the coating to an underlying substrate [345, 440].

A number of primary factors could have an effect on the mechanical reliability of both thin and thick films and coatings according to the work of Nix [467]. Nevertheless, the most crucial factors include residual stresses, substrate roughness, interfacial properties, and the geometry and thickness of the coating.

As previously mentioned, the evaluation of stress in a nanocoating due to deposition technique and heat treatments applied is imperative to its mechanical stability. The successful application of biomaterial implants is largely determined by the likelihood of the coating to crack or spall as a result of external mechanical loading or from inbuilt stresses (whether they are tensile or compressive).

Typically, the most widely used techniques for describing the performance of micro- and nanocoatings on substrates can be categorized into the measurement of: (1) adhesion strength, and (2) coating properties.

Determining the adhesion strength of a coating is vital to ensure that it is properly adhered to the substrate material to which it is applied. As demonstrated by Mittal, a number of techniques have been utilized to measure the adhesive strength of thin films and coatings [468]. The most popular test methods for determining the bond strength between the coating and substrate include indentation scratching at increasing loads, pin-on-disk, and pull-off testing. Other tests such as microtensile tensile are also excellent for determining the adhesion integrity between the micro- and nanocoating and the substrate.

As well as determining the adhesive behavior of coatings, it is also important to evaluate the mechanical properties of thin films and coatings. Consequently, a number of excellent techniques were developed for this purpose and these include scratch testing, tensile testing, bending and bulge testing, nanoindentation, and pull-out test (Table **17**).

Table 17. Summary of the test methods available for evaluating the adhesive or mechanical properties of thin films and coatings.

Test Method	Summary
Scratch Test	Uses an indenter to measures the adhesive strength between a coating and a substrate.
Tensile Pull-Off	Uses tensile stress to separate a coated-test specimen glued to uncoated coupons using structural adhesive. Measures the adhesive strength between a coating and a substrate.
Shear Test	Similar to tensile pull-off. Sufficiently strong bonding agent is required. Measures the adhesive strength between a coating and a substrate.
Bulge and Blister Test	A gas or fluid is used to pressurize the coated specimen. Measures the interfacial energy of coatings to debond from substrate.
In Situ Microtensile Test	Coating is deposited on a tensile coupon. Measures the interfacial delamination between a coating and a substrate.
Bend Delamination Test	Measures the interfacial fracture energy of coatings and thin films.
Instrumented Nanoindentation	Method of choice for determining the mechanical properties of implants and coatings.

13.4.5.1. Scratch Testing

By far the most popular and commonly used method for assessing the adhesive strength between a coating and a substrate (Fig. **41**), the test utilizes a hard diamond or metal spherical tipped indenter with a typical radius of 200 μm. A load is applied through the indenter to the surface of the coating. As the load steadily increases, the specimen is displaced at the same time at a constant speed [469 - 473].

Using microscopy, coating failure can be ascertained from the distance and load from which delamination occurs. It can also be determined using an acoustic emission sensor or from the change in friction. In addition to the critical load, the applied normal force, the tangential (friction) force, and the penetration depth are also obtained.

Scratching of the surface will lead to an escalation in elastic and plastic deformation and at some critical load ($F_{critical}$) widespread spalling of the coating from the substrate will occur. In general, friction force measurements, optical microscopy, or acoustic emissions are used to establish the critical load.

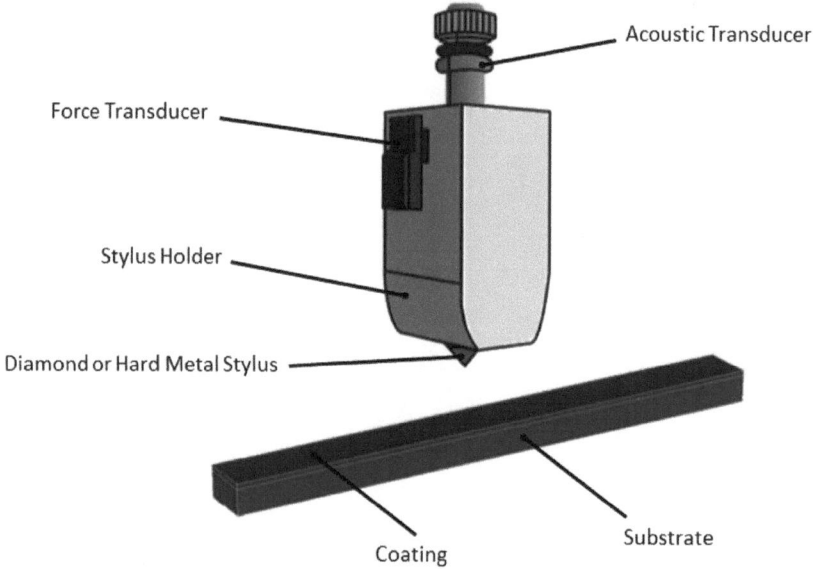

Fig. (41). Illustration showing a typical scratch testing device (based on the Quad Group Inc. Romulus III universal test equipment. ASTM C1624-05: Standard test method for adhesion strength and mechanical failure modes of ceramic coatings by quantitative single point scratch testing.).

The practical work of adhesion (W_{prac}) for a coating on a substrate can be calculated once the critical load ($F_{critical}$) is determined as well as using information such as elastic modulus (E_{coat}), the contact radius (a), and thickness of the coating (t_{coat}) [474, 475]:

$$W_{prac} = \left(\frac{F_{critical}}{\pi a^2}\right)^2 \frac{2t_{coat}}{E_{coat}} \qquad (61)$$

On the other hand, the residual stress in the coating is not taken into consideration in eq. (61). In another similar study [471], the practical work of adhesion for purely elastic coatings on stiff substrates can be described using the following equation:

$$W_{prac} = \frac{\sigma^2 t_{coat}}{2E_{coat}} \qquad (62)$$

In eq. (62), σ is a function in the coating calculated from the residual stress (σ_{res}) and the applied stress (σ_{appl}):

$$\sigma = \sigma_{res} + \sigma_{appl} \tag{63}$$

Yet again, eq. (63) takes into consideration the residual stress (σ_{res}) within the coating, but it is not completely valid for describing the stresses once some plastic deformation transpires. These important studies were further developed so that the residual stress and elastic stress distribution in the coating is considered.

Consequently, an improved equation was derived for calculating the strain energy release rate (γ) using the shear modulus of the coating (G_{coat}), and the average normal (σ_{ij}) and elastic shear (τ_{ij}) stresses in the delaminated coating [476, 477]:

$$\gamma = \left[\frac{(1 - v_{coat}^2)t_{coat}\sigma_{res}^2}{2E_{coat}} \right] + \sum \left[\frac{(1 - v_{coat}^2)t_{coat}\bar{\tau}_{ij}^2}{2G_{coat}} + \frac{(1 - v_{coat}^2)t_{coat}\bar{\sigma}_{ij}^2}{2E_{coat}} \right] \tag{64}$$

In general, scratch testing needs to be handled with extreme care due to the broad array of damage processes that can take place as well as the complex stress states involved. Likewise, the results of scratch testing can be influenced by factors related to the properties of the coating and substrate such as hardness, roughness, and thickness of the coating. In addition, variables such as the loading rate, tip shape, environment and scratching speed also need to be taken into consideration during the test.

13.4.5.2. Tensile Pull-Off and Shear Testing

During tensile pull-off testing, a tensile load applied perpendicular to the coating-substrate interface is used to determine the bonding or adhesive strength between the coating and substrate (Fig. **42**). A structural adhesive is used to glue a coated-test specimen with a typical diameter of 25 mm to an uncoated coupon [478]. The adhesive strength is determined when the coating is separated from the substrate using a tensile force, basically the maximum load over the coated area. Typically, more than five coated coupons are tested, and the averaged adhesion strength is calculated using the test results obtained.

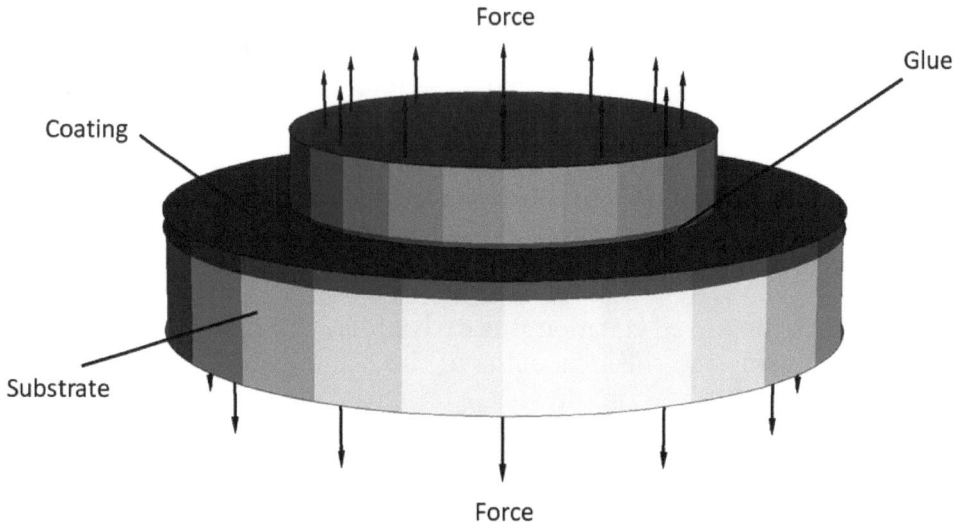

Fig. (42). Illustration showing a typical tensile pull-off test. In the analysis of calcium phosphate coatings, a number of ISO and ASTM standard test methods are available and can be used for design and quality control purposes: ASTM F1147-05 (Standard test method for tension testing of calcium phosphate and metallic coatings.); ISO 13779-4 (Implants for surgery - hydroxyapatite - part 4: determination of coating adhesion strength.); and ASTM C633-01 (Standard test method for adhesion or cohesion strength of thermal spray coatings.).

On the other hand, the shear test method is similar apart from the fact that the load is applied parallel to the interface to the bonded coating layer (Fig. **43**). A relatively strong bonding adhesive is needed in this test to separate the coating from the substrate when shear stress is applied [479].

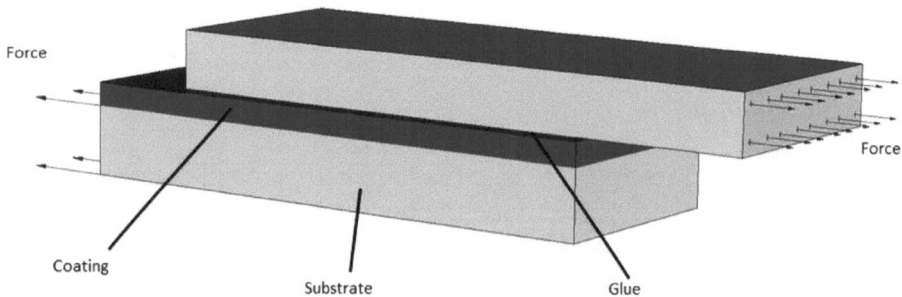

Fig. (43). Illustration showing a typical shear test. In the analysis of calcium phosphate coatings, an ASTM standard test method is available and can be used for design and quality control purposes: ASTM F1044-05 (Standard Test Method for Shear Testing of Calcium Phosphate Coatings and Metallic Coatings.)

The disadvantages associated with these testing methods are related to the pulling of the coating without any misalignment issues in a direction normal or parallel to the interface as well as the consistency during application and the strength of the adhesive used. In addition, if the coating is porous, a diffusion of adhesives may occur resulting in inaccurate or false strength values. Furthermore, the need to visually confirm whether it is adhesive failure or cohesive failure after shear testing is also a concern.

13.4.5.3. Bulge and Blister Test

In the bulge test, a gas or a fluid applied through a hole in the substrate is used to pressurize a coating-substrate system. An interferometer or an optical microscopy is used to measure the height of the resulting hemispherical bulge in the coating. The pressure applied and the deflection height can be used to provide information such as time-dependent, and elastic and plastic deformations.

This is somewhat different to the approach for the blister test. During the test, the pressure is increased until the coating starts to debond from the substrate.

The interfacial energy (γ_{inter}) can be determined from the critical pressure for debonding using the applied pressure (p), radius of the hole (r), and coating properties such as thickness (t_{coat}), elastic modulus (E_{coat}), and Poisson's ratio (v_{coat}) [480]:

$$\gamma_{inter} = \frac{p^2 \, (3 - v_{coat}^2) r^4}{16 E_{coat} t_{coat}^3} \tag{65}$$

13.4.5.4. In Situ Microtensile Test

During microtensile testing, a tensile coupon is used as substrate and a coating is deposited on its surface. It is then pulled using a universal testing machine or a specialized device that can be placed in a scanning electron microscope or under the objective lens of an optical microscope (Fig. **44**). Cracking, damage evolution, and failure in the coating can be observed *in situ* or *ex situ* after the application of specific strains [378, 481 - 484].

Through the application of controlled external stresses, *in situ* microtensile test provides insight into the susceptibility of interfacial delamination between a coating and a substrate. Furthermore, it is also ideal in establishing the properties of both thin and thick coatings on a variety of ductile substrates.

It is also beneficial to tensile test coatings using this method as fairly small test specimens can be used and the stress field is uniform along the gauge length.

During loading, observing the damage *in situ* using scanning electron or optical microscopes can provide useful information into the mechanisms behind material failure [485, 486]. Furthermore, valuable qualitative insights into the susceptibility of a coating to cracking and de-adhesion can be gained by examining the evolution in cracking and debonding during loading. It should be mentioned that when analyzing coating behavior, the residual stress must be determined from substrate curvature measurements, while results obtained from nanoindentation is used to ascertain the elastic modulus of the coating [487].

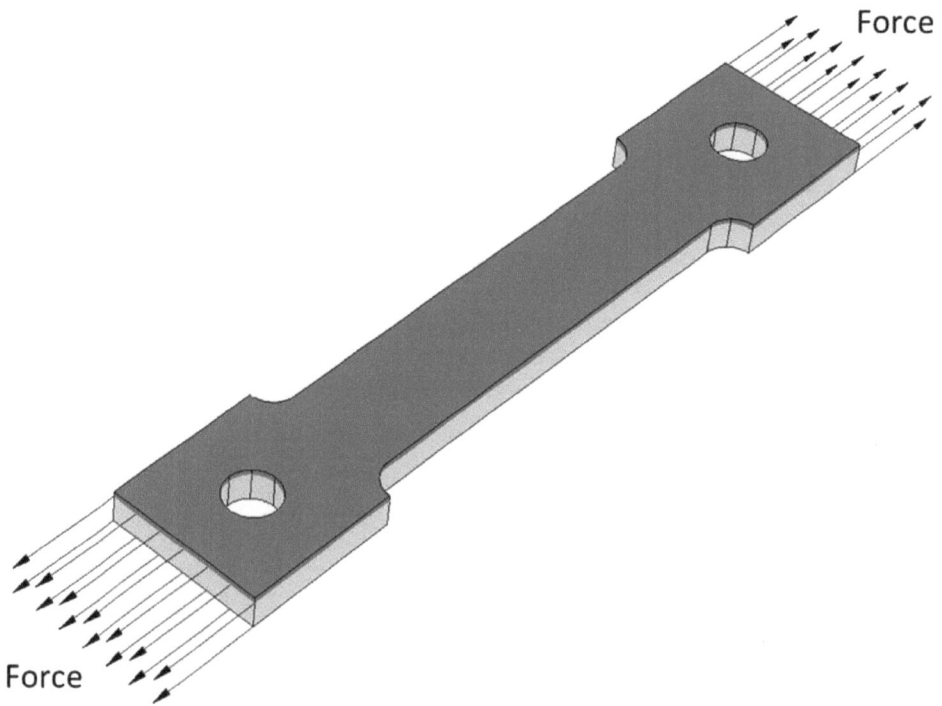

Fig. (44). Illustration showing a coated tensile test specimen pulled during microtensile testing.

Brittle coatings on ductile substrates in most cases, such as calcium phosphate coatings on titanium (Ti-6Al-4V), can produce parallel cracks normal to the tensile axis as soon as it is stressed in the uniaxial direction. As the coated substrate elongates, a reduction in crack spacing is observed due to an increasing amount of these cracks appearing. Significant delamination of the coating can also be caused by the presence of these cracks. For softer and more compliant coatings on the other hand, cracking can be irregular and the likelihood of the coating to debond from the substrate is reduced substantially. The disadvantage with these softer, semi-brittle coatings is the difficulty when it comes to their quantitative analysis.

The coating strength, interface energy, and interfacial shear stress can be determined using fracture mechanics [366]. The critical stress for cracking (σ_{crack}) is calculated using the elastic modulus of the coating (E_{coat}) and the effect of the residual stress (σ_{res}). The residual stress is the result of drying and firing of the coating as well as the variations in the coefficient of thermal expansion between the coating and substrate.

$$\sigma_{crack} = \varepsilon_{crack}E_{coat} + \sigma_{res} \tag{66}$$

As soon as the substrate is strained in tension, ε_{crack} is the instant when cracking first appears in the coating.

Using the value of σ_{crack} determined in eq. (66), the interfacial shear stress (τ_{inter}) can be determined [481]:

$$\tau_{inter} = \frac{\sigma_{crack}t_{coat}\pi}{1.5\lambda} \tag{67}$$

where t_{coat} is the coating thickness and λ is the average crack spacing.

The fracture toughness (K_{IC}) of the coating [483] can be calculated using the yield stress of the substrate material ($\sigma_{sub\text{-}yield}$) and the function of the elastic contrast between the coating and substrate ($F(\alpha_D)$) determined experimentally [488].

$$K_{IC} = \left(\sigma_{crack}^2 t_{coat}\left[\pi F(\alpha_D) + \frac{\sigma_{crack}}{\sqrt{3}\sigma_{sub-yield}}\right]\right)^{\frac{1}{2}} \tag{68}$$

The adhesion between a coating and a substrate can be calculated using the strain (ε_i) measured at the moment when detachment of buckling of the coating is first seen. Once coating delamination takes place, the apparent interfacial fracture energy or the steady state strain energy release rate for a phase angle of approximately 50° is given by [473]:

$$\gamma_{inter} = \frac{1}{2}\varepsilon_i^2 E_{coat}t_{coat} \tag{69}$$

13.4.5.5. Bend Delamination Test

The interfacial fracture between dissimilar materials as well as coatings on substrates has been examined using three- and four-point bending tests. The three-point bend test has been shown to provide an adequate means of determining the interfacial fracture energy of coatings and thin films [489]. The test method is quite straightforward and the test samples can be prepared with relative ease. On the other hand, the results obtained are affected by factors such as the loading geometry, strain rate, and the test sample itself.

Cracks produced adjacent to the coating-substrate interface are required for the test to work from the notch using a simple energy balance for the system prior to cracking and debonding. It also depends on the crucial moment when the crack deflects into and along the interface (Fig. **45**).

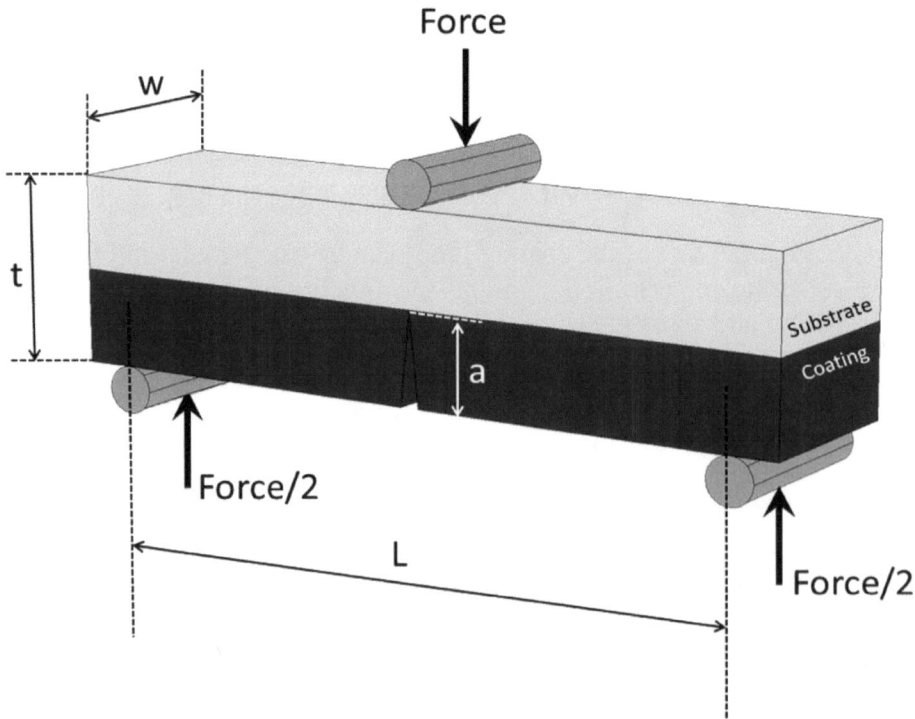

Fig. (45). Illustration showing a three-point bend test.

The test can provide the flexural stress-strain response of the material being tested. The flexural stress ($\sigma_{flexural}$) can be calculated using the load (F) applied at any given point during the test and the length of the support span (L):

$$\sigma_{flexural} = \frac{3FL}{2wt^2} \tag{70}$$

where w and t is the width and thickness of the test specimen, respectively.

On the other hand, the four-point bend test has become a reliable approach for measuring the adhesion of a coating to a metallic substrate (Fig. **46**). A bend bar of the coated substrate with a notch machined in the coated layer is required using this technique as first described by Charalambides *et al.* [490].

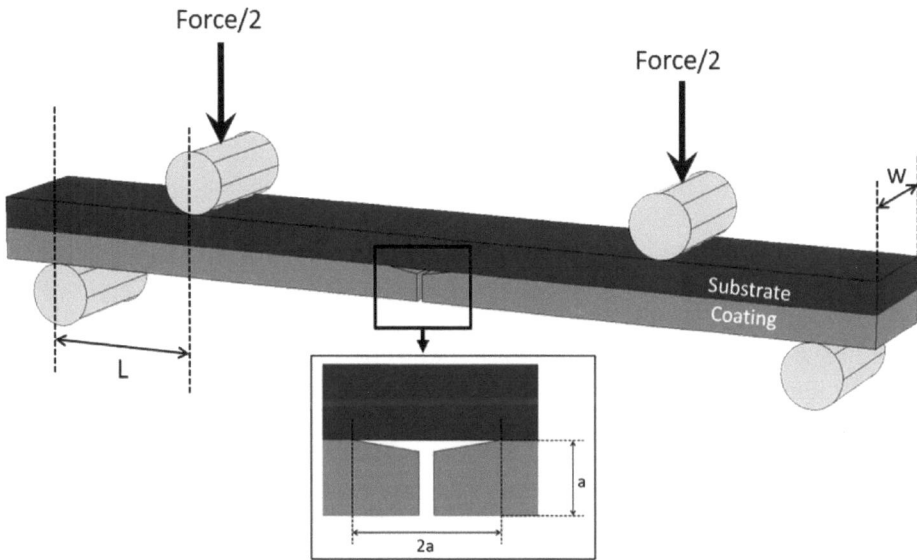

Fig. (46). Schematic of the four-point bend delamination test.

A crack initiates from the notch as the bending moment increases and propagates to the interface. The constant moment condition is defined as the period when the crack deflects and propagates alongside the interface at a critical load. The strain energy release rate (γ), for a phase angle of 41°, can be calculated using:

$$\gamma = \frac{M^2(1 - v_{sub}^2)}{2E_{sub}}\left(\frac{1}{I_{sub}} - \frac{\lambda}{I_{composite}}\right) \tag{71}$$

$$M = \frac{FL}{2w} \tag{72}$$

where F is the plateau load, L is the distance between the inner and outer loading rollers, and w is the width of the test sample (Fig. **46**).

The values of λ, I_{sub}, and $I_{composite}$ can be calculated using the elastic modulus, Poisson's ratio, and the thicknesses of the coating and substrates:

$$\lambda = \frac{E_{sub}(1 - v^2_{coat})}{E_{coat}(1 - v^2_{sub})} \tag{73}$$

$$I_{sub} = \frac{t^3_{sub}}{12} \tag{74}$$

$$I_{composite} = \frac{t^3_{coat}}{12} + \frac{\lambda t^3_{sub}}{12} + \frac{\lambda t_{coat} t_{sub}(t_{coat} + t_{sub})^2}{4(t_{coat} + \lambda t_{sub})} \tag{75}$$

The strain energy release rate is not related to the debond crack length and is a function solely to the critical load for delamination and the specimen geometry.

Four-point bend test, in addition to establishing the strain energy release rate, has also been used to evaluate quantitatively the interfacial fracture energy. The thickness of these substrates is in general much smaller compared to their lateral dimensions. As a result, simple beam bending mechanics can be utilized to determine their elastic response [491].

An approach based on fracture mechanics using four-point bending was developed to measure the interfacial fracture energy at the interface between dissimilar materials [490]. As the bending moment increases, a crack is initiated from the notch, and then it propagates to the interface. For a sufficiently weak interfacial bond, the crack will deflect and propagate along the interface. The interfacial fracture energy ($\gamma_{inter.}$) can be determined using the critical load for stable crack propagation ($F_{critical}$):

$$\gamma = \frac{21L^2 F^2_{critical}(1 - v^2_{sub})}{16 E_{sub} w^2 t^3} \tag{76}$$

The advantage of this method lies in the fact the crack length is unrelated to the interface fracture energy as long as the crack tip is no where near the loading points or the pre-crack.

13.4.5.6. Instrumented Nanoindentation

Nanoindentation testing is the starting point by many dental and biomedical researchers and the method of choice used to ascertain the mechanical properties of implants and coatings. It is now considered a simple and effective method of obtaining important information such as the elastic modulus and hardness of micro- and nanocoatings (Fig. **47**).

In addition to presenting information on the mechanical properties of coatings, nanoindentation testing can also provide a comprehensive assessment of the elastic-plastic response between various coating-substrate combinations (*i.e.* soft/hard and rigid/compliant coating on soft/hard and rigid/compliant substrate) from the loading and unloading curves.

During a typical microindentation test, a load is applied to the material surface *via* a diamond tip with a known geometry, normally Knoop, Rockwell, or Vickers. The area of the residual impression is determined once the load is removed using optical means. This residual impression is then used to determine the hardness of the material. On the other hand, the size of the residual impression in nanoindentation testing is often only a few microns, obtaining a direct measurement utilizing optical approaches are extremely challenging.

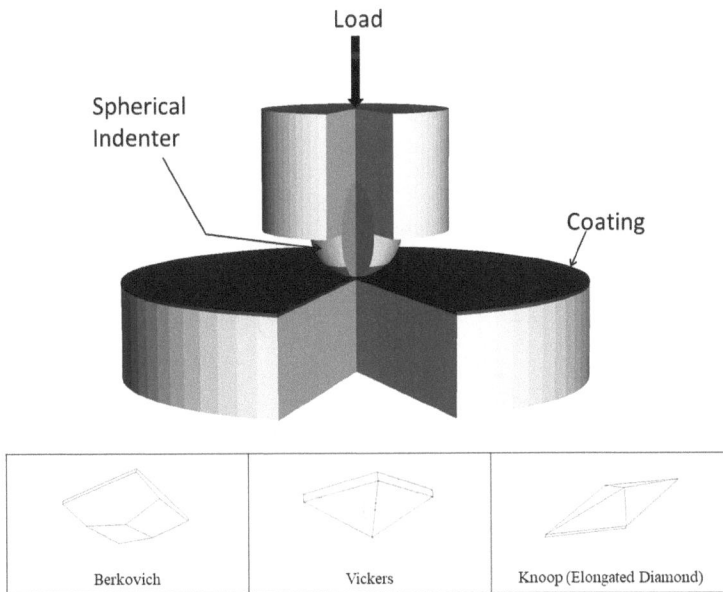

Fig. (47). Schematic of a nanoindentation test using a spherical indenter (Brinell Hardness Test). Other available indenters are also shown.

During nanoindentation testing, a set load in milli-newtons is applied to the indenter resting on top of the specimen. As the load is applied, the penetration depth in nanometers is then measured. The mean contact pressure or hardness is obtained by dividing the maximum load (F) over the project contact area (A) which is determined using the indenter geometry and the contact depth [492]:

$$H = \frac{F}{A} \tag{77}$$

The radius or known angle of the indenter together with the depth of impression are used to calculate the area of contact at maximum load (Fig. **47**).

The result of a nanoindentation test is displayed in the form of a load-displacement curve (Fig. **48**). Information that can be obtained from the graph includes contact pressure or hardness and the elastic modulus of the test sample using the slope of the curve during unloading along with software based on the model and the type of indenter used, such as Brinell, Vickers, Knoop, or Berkovich [437, 492 - 494]. Likewise, various types of loading and unloading techniques can be used to extract required properties as a function of penetration depth.

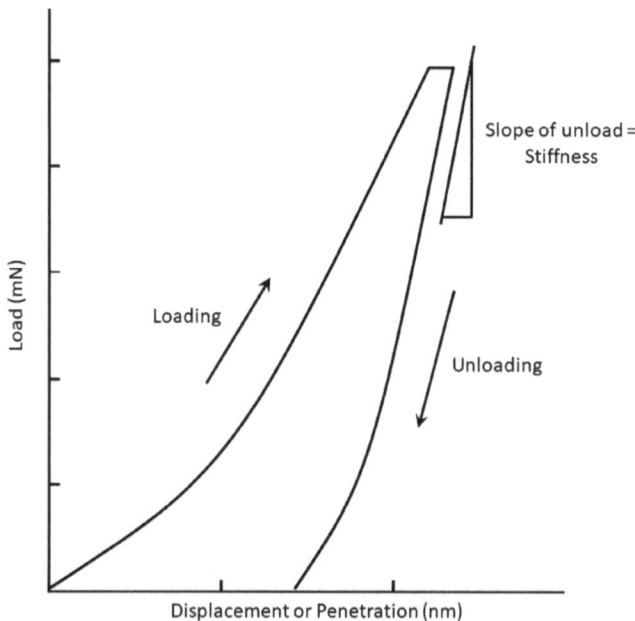

Fig. (48). A load-displacement graph obtained from a nanoindentation test.

The elastic modulus (E) can be calculated using the slope or gradient of the curve during unloading, which is also known as contact stiffness, as shown in Fig. (**48**):

$$Contact\ Stiffness = \frac{\Delta\ load}{\Delta\ penetration} = \frac{2}{\sqrt{\pi}}E\sqrt{A} \tag{78}$$

where A is the area obtained at maximum load.

It is worthy to mention that eq. (78) is valid for elastic contacts using axis-symmetric indenters such spherical, conical, and cylindrical punches.

The combined elastic modulus of the indenter and specimen (E_{com}) can be determined using the following equation:

$$\frac{1}{E_{com}} = \frac{(1 - v_{ind}^2)}{E_{ind}} + \frac{(1 - v_{spec}^2)}{E_{spec}} \tag{79}$$

The accuracy of the result from nanoindentation testing is dependent on factors such as sample preparation, calibration of equipment, indenter tip shape, initial penetration, frame compliance, and corrections for thermal drift [492 - 494].

Nanoindentation can also be applied towards determining coating adhesion and residual stress from transverse scratching or direct indentation, as previously described by Fischer-Cripps [494]. Furthermore, nanoindenters in particular, have also been utilized to measure residual stress and coating adhesion to the substrate obtained from the load that resulted in delamination taken from the "pop-in" that corresponds to a discontinuity or a plateau in the load-displacement curve (Fig. **48**). In the same way, the creep and viscoelastic behavior of soft materials can be investigated. This is extremely relevant to researches in bone and biological tissue studies and in dental resins and composites.

13.4.5.7. Finite Element Indentation Testing

The use of FEA has been widely adopted by materials and biomedical researchers for studying the response of a material when subjected to a micro- and nanoindentation test, and in particular, the elastic and plastic behaviors beneath a pointed indenter (Fig. **49**).

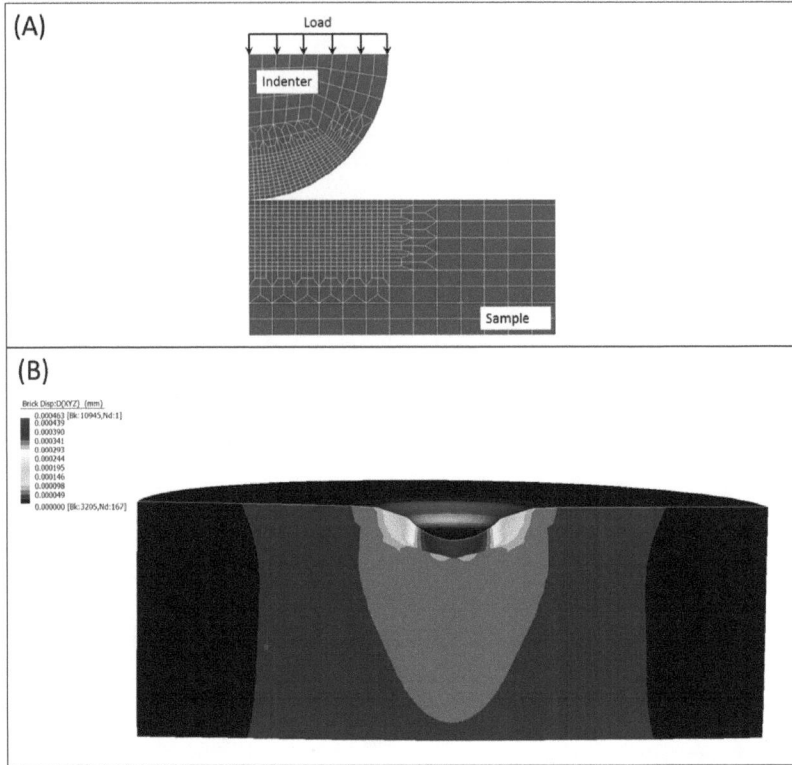

Fig. (49). Simple illustration of a three-dimensional FEA indentation testing model. (**A**) The load is applied to the top of the indenter that is resting on the surface of the test specimen. The base of the substrate is fixed to prevent movement during simulation; (**B**) Deformation of the test specimen at the conclusion of the nanoindentation simulation.

Numerous benefits are offered by FEA, for instance a reduction in the experimental time and the relative ease in altering the physical and mechanical properties of a coating-substrate system, such as the thickness and elastic properties. Large-scale commercial codes are available at the moment for FEA software which provides a simulation atmosphere for various indenter tips, substrates, and coatings. Through the combined efforts of experimental data on indentation and FEA will provide better knowledge regarding the fracture and deformation of coatings, in addition to expanding our awareness into the mechanical characteristics of thin film/coating-substrate system.

The application of FEA to examine the indentation process on a number of coatings such as diamond-like carbon (DLC), titanium nitride (TiN), and zirconia using spherical indenters has been extensively investigated since the late 1990s. Furthermore, studies were also conducted using other indenter tips such as

Berkovich and Vickers [440].

The interfacial adhesions of a coating-substrate system under indentation have also been examined using FEA. A study was carried out in 2007 to examine the interfacial delamination and buckling of thin films subjected to micro-wedge indentation [495]. Their model assumed the interface connecting the thin film and substrate is the only local in which cracking can occur. The failure and adhesive characteristics at the interface separating the thin film and substrate was simulated using a traction-separation law with interface energy and strength as the two primary parameters.

13.4.5.8. Finite Element Adhesion Testing

In addition to simulating the indentation process, investigations were also conducted to examine the adhesion and debonding process of coatings. In a previous study, the adhesion and debonding process of thin films were described using a non-linear beam formula which takes into account the adhesion caused by surface tractions and by body forces [496]. The hypothesized beam formula was validated against both analytical peeling models and currently available two- and three-dimensional solid FEA models.

In another study, a geometrically non-linear two-dimensional plain strain finite element model was constructed to examine the deformation behavior of thin films under simulated pull-off test [497]. Their results revealed an agreement exists between the theoretical constitutive relation and the strain energy release rate and the results obtained from FEA simulation at different residual stress levels, which played a critical role in both the constitutive relation and the energy release rate. Later, a three-dimensional finite element model was constructed to examine the interfacial delamination between a thin film strop and a stiff substrate during a pull-off test. They suggested that a three-dimensional model is able to provide a deeper insight into the delamination process, information that cannot be attained in their earlier study [498].

CONCLUDING REMARKS

Acquiring a deeper insight into the manufacturing process in addition to the properties of bioceramics (physical, mechanical, and biological) currently used as implants and as bone replacement materials could significantly contribute to the design of new-generation prostheses and implantable devices as well as post-operative patient management policies.

The advantages of utilizing advanced ceramic materials in dental and oral and maxillofacial applications have generally been welcomed, and in particularly in terms of their biocompatibility and strength. Enhancements in the fabrication process, for instance the application of hot isostatic pressing, can produce ceramic materials with higher densities and smaller grain structures which are essential for their utilizations in dentistry, oral and maxillofacial surgery, and in biomedical applications. Furthermore, the combination of very fine grain structure and the use of suitable sintering aids will allow the fabrication of ceramics with a density close to its theoretical values, and this will result in the optimization of strength in addition to preventing propagation of cracks and ultimately the fracture of the material.

At present, alumina and partially stabilized zirconia ceramics are used in dental implants as well as in maxillofacial surgery with great success. Moreover, the utilization of bioglasses as body-interactive materials is of critical importance in the restoration of physiological functions by assisting the body to promote the regeneration of tissues or to heal. The application of bioglasses can be further explored in the development of next-generation bioactive glasses that can incorporate biogenic materials and specific drugs, which are intended to enhance their functionality and capabilities.

The ideal material of choice when considering a bone replacement would be synthetic calcium phosphate as it can mimic the composition and structure of the bone mineral HAp. The birth of nanotechnology has created novel approaches for the production of synthetic bone-like calcium phosphate nanopowders and nanocoatings. Without a doubt, the availability of calcium phosphate nanomaterials has generated new opportunities for the development of superior biocompatible coatings for implants and high-strength dental nanocomposites. On the other hand, the mechanical properties of calcium phosphate are far from being close to those of human bone despite having a similar chemistry and composition. This can be resolved through the creation of a nanocomposite by combining calcium phosphate with other micro- and nanoscale materials as a secondary phase.

Dental and oral and maxillofacial implants used primarily for tooth replacement and fracture fixation include ceramic and metallic (and to a certain extent polymeric materials) screws, plates, nails and implants. These implants are of vital importance because they facilitate an adequate attachment to bone and display the required mechanical properties including strength, elasticity, ductility and necessary wear resistance. At the bone-implant interface, the stiffness of the implant material used will govern the amount of load it can carry. For instance, the stiffness of titanium or zirconia allows it to endure greater loads or force than compared to the surrounding bone tissues that have a much lower stiffness values. This imbalance in load, which is also referred to as stress shielding, can result in the resorption of bone tissue. More importantly, an implant that is too stiff or rigid may also increase the possibility of bone fracture. This is the consequence of the bone becoming thinned or osteoporotic as a result of excessive protection created by the stress shielding effect of the implant. By using the composite approach, it is possible to design the composite with mechanical properties such as elastic modulus and strength much closer to those of natural bone, through the help of secondary substitution phases. This will reduce the effect of stress shielding caused by a mismatch in mechanical properties between human bone and the implant material used.

Biomaterials in nature are produced through self-assembly into highly organized structures from energy efficient and immaculate resource using common and readily available substrates. Functional structures optimized to their environment are manufactured using this approach. Gaining an understanding of the way natural materials are made and the way these materials adapt to their environment will allow us to synthesize an exciting collection of self-responsive structures and materials that can be used in regenerative medicine. This will also provide us with the opportunity to synthesize structures using nanocoatings and nanocomposite structures with intricate architectures and shapes that are tailored to their functions and with a very slim chance of failure.

The use of biomimetic approach can produce promising outcomes for applications in tissue engineering of skeletal tissues. One such approach involves the reconfiguration of the material environments at the molecular and macromolecular level that attempt to mimic native extracellular matrix. The aim is to further expand this approach towards designing clinically relevant scaffolds that can be used in regenerative medicine. This can be achieved through the utilization of self-organizing hierarchical structures created and produced based on biological principles of design. Meanwhile, advanced functional biomaterials and nanobiomaterials are being constructed by controlling inorganic molecules, nanoparticles and nanocoatings with enormous precision by harnessing the power of nature that can be utilized in tissue engineering as well as pharmaceutical drug and gene delivery.

In the next decade, there will be an increase in the application of implants, prostheses and devices containing nanocoatings and nanocomposite coatings. The relationship between the biological responses of materials and their surface properties is a major question that needs to be addressed in biomaterials research. Surface modification using nanocoatings and nanocomposite coatings has become a vital tool in the research aimed at gaining an insight into how the chemical and surface properties of the materials used will influence its interaction with the biological system. As a deeper understanding is achieved, it is anticipated that surface modifications aimed at controlling tissue response will generate new opportunities for the research and development of new and improved dental and oral and maxillofacial implants and prostheses in a more rapid and systemic manner. However, the issue of surface interactions will get more complicated in a changing world where implants and prostheses will be modified not only by biomaterials such as calcium phosphate but also with bisphosphonates and biogenic materials such as bone morphogenetic proteins, peptides, growth factors, as well as by a variety of stem cells such as mesenchymal stem cells. Furthermore, standardizing test results between different biomaterials would be difficult due to its morphology being heterogeneous.

Undoubtedly, the complications most frequently associated with the use of implantable medical devices such as dental implants are bacterial infections. In order to alleviate the problem associated with biofilm infections, several strategies have been suggested based on either preventing and/or controlling bacterial infections. A promising approach in the prevention of device-related infections is the development of multifunctional nanocoatings and nanocomposite coatings with surface properties that have an effect against microbial viability or adhesion. Another method is to alter the surface of medical devices biologically, physically, and chemically to render the surface free of microbial adhesion.

The search is ongoing to find a more effective and less costly means of delivering antibiotics to fight against bacterial infections without the complications associated with long-term intravenous access and the toxicity of systemic antibiotics. For any drug carriers that utilize nanocoatings and nanocomposite coatings, the appropriate rates of dissolution as well as their control within the human body is the primary concern. A number of studies were carried out to investigate ways in which long-term release or long circulating time carriers can be developed. Among these, the surface modification of nanocoatings and nanocomposite coatings with a variety of polymeric macromolecules or nonionic surfactant were found to be the most effective. Nevertheless, appropriate and efficient modifications of the nanoparticles within multifunctional nanocoatings are a necessity for the future for slow drug delivery devices and systems. Research in the future will focus on disabling biofilm resistance by deactivating certain genes of bacteria that are responsible for antibiotic resistance in a process known as gene editing. This may enhance the ability of existing antibiotics to treat infections involving biofilms. A surface that would hinder the biofilm formation or prevent the pathogenic bacteria colonization through anti-biofilm or anti-bacterial agents would constitute a major improvement in the long-term survival of the implants.

New generations of medical implants and devices with these functionalized surfaces will require nanoscale surface properties measuring techniques that can be used to describe both living tissues and inorganic materials as well as the interfacial reactions between implant and bone tissue for future modelling and implant and prosthesis design. The use of theoretical modeling approaches such as FEA is becoming a necessity in the fields of medicine and dentistry. By examining the mechanics of a single cell using FEA, we could potentially accelerate discoveries in the fields of regenerative medicine, drug discovery, and mechanobiology.

More importantly, the use of FEA will have innumerable applications in both dentistry and oral and maxillofacial surgery at a clinical level. The integration of medical imaging technologies such as computed tomography with FEA in the development of accurate patient-matched (or patient specific) three-dimension model will permit clinicians to best address the engineering requirements of implants and prostheses utilized to treat mandibular and maxilla fractures with the intention of attaining both fixation and reduction of the fracture and at the same time minimizing osteosynthesis plate size and number. Computational models of the fracture healing process may prove useful in determining the optimal mechanical-based treatments after an accident or a fall. Nevertheless, we need to consider the difference between nature and FEA simulations. For instance, bone healing is governed by biological, chemical, and genetic factors in addition to being regulated by mechanical factors. These issues need to be addressed in order to improve the predictive accuracy of the bone fracture healing process.

Bone remodeling around various options for tooth restoration can be investigated under functional movements and any potential issues such as stress shielding eliminated by proper surgical protocol, implant design, appropriate guides and navigation system prior to implantation. In addition to biological factors, bone-implant interactions are affected by functionally applied multiaxial forces and biomechanics. The ultimate understanding of biological systems can only be achieved through appropriate nanoscale mechanical properties of biogenic structures and the influence of the nanostructures and nano loading on these biological systems.

Measuring and determining the mechanical properties of nanomaterials using FEA will inevitably generate new avenues in understanding the relationship between stresses and deformations (both micro- and nanoscale) and the growth and repair mechanisms of biologic systems. This knowledge will enable us to employ new materials, tools, and systems in tissue regeneration.

GLOSSARY

DEFINITIONS AND ABBREVIATIONS

Berkovich: A three-sided pyramid with a half angle of 65.27° that is used in nanoindentation testing. It has been estimated that this nanoindenter tip possesses the same area-to-depth ratio as compared to the Vickers indenter.

Bite: Bite Force.

Brinell Hardness Test: This hardness test utilizes a hard spherical indenter which is pressed into the surface of the test material under a standard load.

coat: Coating.

Compressive Strength: The maximum stress a material can withstand in compression without fracture.

Creep: Time-dependent permanent deformation of a material when subjected to a constant load. Creep is an important issue for most materials at elevated temperatures.

CT: Computed Tomography.

Elastic Deformation: Non-permanent deformation. Material totally recovers upon the release of the applied stress or load.

Elastic Modulus (E): Also referred to as the stiffness, Young's modulus or modulus of elasticity. It is a measure of how stiff or flexible a material is, *i.e.* the higher the E value, the stiffer the material. Typically expressed in GPa (gigapascal). 1 GPa = 1×10^9 Pa.

ext: External Pterygoid Muscle.

F: Force or Load.

FEA: Finite Element Analysis.

FEM: Finite Element Modelling.

Fracture Toughness (K_{IC}): A quantitative way of describing a material's resistance to brittle fracture when a crack is present. The key in using fracture toughness in design is to select a material with a high K_{IC} as it can tolerate higher stress and/or larger crack size.

HAp: Hydroxyapatite.

Hardness (H): Defined as the ability of a material to resist indentation penetration, abrasion, and scratching. The most commonly used hardness testing techniques include Rockwell, Knoop, Vickers, and Brinell.

iEMG: Integrated Electromyography.

ind: Indenter.

int: Internal Pterygoid Muscle.

inter: Interface.

Knoop Microhardness Test: Similar to Vickers Microhardness Test. An elongated diamond indenter is used instead. Primarily used to examine the hardness of brittle materials such as ceramics.

mass: Masseter Muscle.

nm: Nanometer or 1×10^{-9} m.

Plastic Deformation: Opposite to elastic deformation. Deformation is non-recoverable or permanent after the applied stress or load is released.

Poisson's ratio (v): Characterizes the contraction perpendicular to the extension caused by a tensile stress.

Rockwell Hardness Test: The simplest and the most common technique for measuring the hardness of materials. A standard spherical or conical indenter is forced into the material under a known dead load. The material to be tested will determine which Rockwell hardness scale is used. Hence, both the hardness value and the scale used must be included when specifying Rockwell hardness.

Shear Modulus (G): Also known as modulus of rigidity. It can be defined as the response of a material to shear stress and it is determined from the gradient of a shear stress-strain graph (the linear elastic portion).

Shear Strain (γ): Described as the tangent of the shear angle which is caused by an applied shear load.

Shear Stress (τ): Can be described as the components of stresses that act parallel to a given plane.

spec: Specimen.

Strain (ε): Defined as the change per unit length in a linear dimension; it is a dimensionless quantity (*i.e.* no units).

Strain Energy: Described as the work done in distorting a body by the application of an external force. This work or energy is stored in the body if the elastic limit is not exceeded and this energy is referred to as strain energy.

Stress (σ): Defined as the distribution of internal force per unit area within the specimen. Typically expressed in Pa (pascal) or MPa (megapascal). 1 MPa 1×10^6 Pa.

SED: Strain Energy Density.

sub: Substrate.

t: Thickness.

temp: Temporalis Muscle.

TMJ: Temporomandibular Joint.

Tensile Strength: The maximum stress a material can withstand in tension without fracture.

Toughness: It is a measure of energy needed to break a unit volume of material. It is approximated by the area under the stress-strain graph.

Vickers Microhardness Test: Utilizes a square diamond pyramid indenter to measure the hardness of a material when it is pressed into the surface using a load smaller than what is used in Brinell and Rockwell Hardness Test.

Viscoelasticity: a form of deformation displaying the mechanical qualities of elastic deformation and viscous flow.

w: Width.

Yield Stress: It is the stress at which a material begins to plastically deform. If a material is subjected to a stress level that is below the yield stress, it will deform elastically and it will return to its original size and dimension once the applied stress is removed.

γ: Energy.

ρ: Density.

σ_{appl}: Applied Stress.

σ_{res}: Residual Stress.

μm: Micrometer or 1×10^{-6} m, also referred to as micron.

REFERENCES

[1]   Hudis MM. The mouth; medical considerations in the construction and design of oral prostheses. Ann Dent 1978; 37(2): 45-56.[PMID: 354476]

[2]   Atkinson PJ, Woodhead C. Remodeling in the aging mandible--a factor in implant dentistry. J Oral Implantol 1979; 8(3): 353-70.[PMID: 297792]

[3]   Schnitman PA, Shulman LB. Dental implants--their current status. J Mass Dent Soc 1977; 26(4): 278-86.[PMID: 273649]

[4]   Albrektsson T, Sennerby L. State of the art in oral implants. J Clin Periodontol 1991; 18(6): 474-81.[http://dx.doi.org/10.1111/j.1600-051X.1991.tb02319.x] [PMID: 1890231]

[5]   Palmer R. Introduction to dental implants. Br Dent J 1999; 187(3): 127-32.[PMID: 10481363]

[6]   Palmer R, Palmer P, Floyd P. Basic implant surgery. Br Dent J 1999; 187(8): 415-21.[PMID: 10716000]

[7]   Palmer R, Howe L. Dental implants. 3. Assessment of the dentition and treatment options for the replacement of missing teeth. Br Dent J 1999; 187(5): 247-55.[PMID: 10520543]

[8]   Palmer P, Palmer R. Dental implants. 8. Implant surgery to overcome anatomical difficulties. Br Dent J 1999; 187(10): 532-40.[PMID: 10630042]

[9]   Skalak R. Biomechanical considerations in osseointegrated prostheses. J Prosthet Dent 1983; 49(6): 843-8.[http://dx.doi.org/10.1016/0022-3913(83)90361-X] [PMID: 6576140]

[10]   Albrektsson T, Zarb G, Worthington P, Eriksson AR. The long-term efficacy of currently used dental implants: a review and proposed criteria of success. Int J Oral Maxillofac Implants 1986; 1(1): 11-25.[PMID: 3527955]

[11]   Grenoble DE. Design criteria for dental implants. Oral Implantol 1974; 5(1): 44-64.[PMID: 4610465]

[12]   Haack JE, Sakaguchi RL, Sun T, Coffey JP. Elongation and preload stress in dental implant abutment screws. Int J Oral Maxillofac Implants 1995; 10(5): 529-36.[PMID: 7590997]

[13]   Rangert BR, Sullivan RM, Jemt TM. Load factor control for implants in the posterior partially edentulous segment. Int J Oral Maxillofac Implants 1997; 12(3): 360-70.[PMID: 9197101]

[14]   Polland KE, Munro S, Reford G, *et al.* The mandibular canal of the edentulous jaw. Clin Anat 2001; 14(6): 445-52.[http://dx.doi.org/10.1002/ca.1080] [PMID: 11754239]

[15]   Duckworth T. Lecture notes on orthopaedic and fractures. Blackwell Scientific Publications, 1980.

[16]   Rodan GA, Bourret LA, Harvey A, Mensi T. Cyclic AMP and cyclic GMP: mediators of the mechanical effects on bone remodeling. Science 1975; 189(4201): 467-469 .[http://dx.doi.org/10.1126/science.168639] [PMID: 168639]

[17]   Binderman I, Shimshoni Z, Somjen D. Biochemical pathways involved in the translation of physical stimulus into biological message. Calcif Tissue Int 1984; 36 (Suppl. 1): S82-S85 .[http://dx.doi.org/10.1007/BF02406139] [PMID: 6331615]

[18]   Katz JL. Hard tissue as a composite material. I. Bounds on the elastic behavior. J Biomech 1971; 4(5): 455-73.[http://dx.doi.org/10.1016/0021-9290(71)90064-9] [PMID: 5133361]

[19]   Katz JL. The structure and biomechanics of bone. In: Vincent JFV, Currey JD, Eds. Mechanical Properties of Biological Materials. Cambridge, Cambridge University Press, 1980; pp. 137-68.

[20]   Piekarski K. Analysis of bone as a composite material. Int J Eng Sci 1973; 11: 557-565 .[http://dx.doi.org/10.1016/0020-7225(73)90018-9]

[21]   Weiss L. Histology: cell and tissue biology. New York, Elsevier Biomedical, 1983; pp 43.

[22]   Robinson RA. Crystal, collagen, and water relationships in bone matrix. Clin Orthop 1960; (17): 69-76.

[23]   Timmins PA, Wall JC. Bone water. Calcif Tissue Res 1977; 23(1): 1-5 .[http://dx.doi.org/10.1007/BF02012759] [PMID: 890540]

[24]   Park JB. Biomaterials: an introduction. New York, Plenum, 1979.

[25]   Katz JL. Anisotropy of Young's modulus of bone. Nature 1980; 283(5742): 106-107 .[http://dx.doi.org/10.1038/283106a0] [PMID: 7350519]

[26]   Lakes R. Materials with structural hierarchy. Nature 1993; 361: 511-515 .[http://dx.doi.org/10.1038/361511a0]

[27]   Frasca P, Harper RA, Katz JL. Scanning electron microscopy studies of collagen, mineral and ground substance in human cortical bone. Scan Electron Microsc 1981; 3(Pt 3): 339-46.[PMID: 7330582]

[28]   Amprino R. Investigations on some physical properties of bone tissue. Acta Anat (Basel) 1958; 34(3): 161-86.[http://dx.doi.org/10.1159/000141381] [PMID: 13594070]

[29]   Evans GP, Behiri JC, Currey JD, Bonfield W. Microhardness and Young's modulus in cortical bone exhibiting a wide range of mineral volume fractions, and in a bone analogue. J Mater Sci Mater Med 1990; 1: 38-43.[http://dx.doi.org/10.1007/BF00705352]

[30]   Rho JY, Tsui TY, Pharr GM. Elastic properties of human cortical and trabecular lamellar bone measured by nanoindentation. Biomaterials 1997; 18(20): 1325-1330 .[http://dx.doi.org/10.1016/S0142-9612(97)00073-2] [PMID: 9363331]

[31]   Turner CH, Rho J, Takano Y, Tsui TY, Pharr GM. The elastic properties of trabecular and cortical bone tissues are similar: results from two microscopic measurement techniques. J Biomech 1999; 32(4): 437-41.[http://dx.doi.org/10.1016/S0021-9290(98)00177-8] [PMID: 10213035]

[32]   Roy ME, Rho JY, Tsui TY, Evans ND, Pharr GM. Mechanical and morphological variation of the human lumbar vertebral cortical and trabecular bone. J Biomed Mater Res 1999; 44(2): 191-7.[http://dx.doi.org/10.1002/(SICI)1097-4636(199902)44:2<191::AID-JBM9>3.0.CO;2-G] [PMID: 10397920]

[33]   Zysset PK, Guo XE, Hoffler CE, Moore KE, Goldstein SA. Elastic modulus and hardness of cortical and trabecular bone lamellae measured by nanoindentation in the human femur. J Biomech 1999; 32(10): 1005-12.[http://dx.doi.org/10.1016/S0021-9290(99)00111-6] [PMID: 10476838]

[34]   Swadener JG, Rho JY, Pharr GM. Effects of anisotropy on elastic moduli measured by nanoindentation in human tibial cortical bone. J Biomed Mater Res 2001; 57(1): 108-12.[http://dx.doi.org/10.1002/1097-4636(200110)57:1<108::AID-JBM1148>3.0.CO;2-6] [PMID: 11416856]

[35]   Fan Z, Rho JY. Effects of viscoelasticity and time-dependent plasticity on nanoindentation measurements of human cortical bone. J Biomed Mater Res A 2003; 67(1): 208-14.[http://dx.doi.org/10.1002/jbm.a.10027] [PMID: 14517878]

[36]   Kim DG, Jeong YH, Kosel E, *et al.* Regional variation of bone tissue properties at the human mandibular condyle. Bone 2015; 77: 98-106.[http://dx.doi.org/10.1016/j.bone.2015.04.024] [PMID: 25913634]

[37]   Waters NE. Some mechanical physical properties of teeth.Mech Prop Biol Mat 1980; 99-134.

[38]   Currey JD. The mechanical consequences of variation in the mineral content of bone. J Biomech 1969; 2(1): 1-11.[http://dx.doi.org/10.1016/0021-9290(69)90036-0] [PMID: 16335107]

[39]   Currey JD. The effects of strain rate, reconstruction and mineral content on some mechanical properties of bovine bone. J Biomech 1975; 8(1): 81-86 .[http://dx.doi.org/10.1016/0021-9290(75)90046-9] [PMID: 1126977]

[40]   Currey JD. The effect of porosity and mineral content on the Young's modulus of elasticity of compact bone. J Biomech 1988; 21(2): 131-9.[http://dx.doi.org/10.1016/0021-9290(88)90006-1] [PMID: 3350827]

[41]   Pernelle K, Imbert L, Bosser C, *et al.* Microscale mechanical and mineral heterogeneity of human cortical bone governs osteoclast activity. Bone 2017; 94: 42-49 .[http://dx.doi.org/10.1016/j.bone.2016.10.002] [PMID: 27725316]

[42]   Hayes WC, Carter DR. Postyield behavior of subchondral trabecular bone. J Biomed Mater Res 1976; 10(4): 537-44.[http://dx.doi.org/10.1002/jbm.820100409] [PMID: 947917]

[43]   Weaver JK, Chalmers J. Cancellous bone: its strength and changes with ageing and an evaluation of some methods for measuring content – I. Age changes in cancellous bone. J Bone Jt Surg 1966; 48a: 289-98.[http://dx.doi.org/10.2106/00004623-196648020-00007]

[44]   Whitehouse WJ, Dyson ED, Jackson CK. The scanning electron microscope in studies of trabecular bone from a human vertebral body. J Anat 1971; 108(Pt 3): 481-96.[PMID: 4930228]

[45]   Carter DR, Hayes WC. The compressive behavior of bone as a two-phase porous material. J Bone Jt Surg 1977; 49: 954-62.[http://dx.doi.org/10.2106/00004623-197759070-00021]

[46]   Williams JL, Lewis JL. Properties and an anisotropic model of cancellous bone from the proximal tibial epiphysis. J Biomech Eng 1982; 104(1): 50-6.[http://dx.doi.org/10.1115/1.3138303] [PMID: 7078118]

[47]   Bensusan JS, Davy DT, Heiple KG, Verdin PJ. Tensile, compressive and torsional testing of cancellous bone. Trans Orth Res Soc 29th Meeting 1983; 132.

[48]   Gibson LJ. The mechanical behaviour of cancellous bone. J Biomech 1985; 18(5): 317-28.[http://dx.doi.org/10.1016/0021-9290(85)90287-8] [PMID: 4008502]

[49]   Müller R, Rüegsegger P. Analysis of mechanical properties of cancellous bone under conditions of simulated bone atrophy. J Biomech 1996; 29(8): 1053-1060 .[http://dx.doi.org/10.1016/0021-9290(96)00006-1] [PMID: 8817372]

[50]   Zioupos P, Cook RB, Hutchinson JR. Some basic relationships between density values in cancellous and cortical bone. J Biomech 2008; 41(9): 1961-8.[http://dx.doi.org/10.1016/j.jbiomech.2008.03.025] [PMID: 18501911]

[51]   Knets IV, Pfafrod GO, Saulgozis JZ. Deformation and fracture of hard biological tissue. Zinatne Riga 1980; 319.

[52]   Ashman RB, Cowin SC, Van Buskirk WC, Rice JC. A continuous wave technique for the measurement of the elastic properties of cortical bone. J Biomech 1984; 17(5): 349-61.[http://dx.doi.org/10.1016/0021-9290(84)90029-0] [PMID: 6736070]

[53]   Ashman RB, Rosinia G, Cowin SC, Fontenot MG, Rice JC. The bone tissue of the canine mandible is elastically isotropic. J Biomech 1985; 18(9): 717-721 .[http://dx.doi.org/10.1016/0021-9290(85)90026-0] [PMID: 4077867]

[54]   Ashman RB, Van Buskirk WC. The elastic properties of a human mandible. Adv Dent Res 1987; 1(1): 64-7.[http://dx.doi.org/10.1177/08959374870010011401] [PMID: 3326617]

[55]   Nail GA, Dechow PC, Ashman RB. Elastic properties of mandibular bone in rhesus monkeys. J Dent Res 1989; 68: 294.

[56]   Dechow PC, Schwartz-Dabney CL, Ashman RB. Elastic properties of the human mandibular corpus. In: Goldstein SA, Carlson DS, Eds. Bone Biodynamics on Orthodontic and Orthopaedic Treatment. Craniofacial growth series. Michigan, University of Michigan, 1992; 27: 299-314.

[57]   Dechow PC, Nail GA, Schwartz-Dabney CL, Ashman RB. Elastic properties of human supraorbital and mandibular bone. Am J Phys Anthropol 1993; 90(3): 291-306 .[http://dx.doi.org/10.1002/ajpa.1330900304] [PMID: 8460653]

[58] Rho JY. An ultrasonic method for measuring the elastic properties of human tibial cortical and cancellous bone. Ultrasonics 1996; 34(8): 777-83.[http://dx.doi.org/10.1016/S0041-624X(96)00078-9] [PMID: 9010460]

[59] Schwartz-Dabney CL, Dechow PC. Variations in cortical material properties from throughout the human mandible. J Dent Res 1997; 76: 249.

[60] Peterson J, Dechow PC. Material properties of the inner and outer cortical tables of the human parietal bone. Anat Rec 2002; 268(1): 7-15.[http://dx.doi.org/10.1002/ar.10131] [PMID: 12209560]

[61] Pithioux M, Lasaygues P, Chabrand P. An alternative ultrasonic method for measuring the elastic properties of cortical bone. J Biomech 2002; 35(7): 961-8.[http://dx.doi.org/10.1016/S0021-9290(02)00027-1] [PMID: 12052398]

[62] Mahmoud A, Cortes D, Abaza A, *et al.* Noninvasive assessment of human jawbone using ultrasonic guided waves. IEEE Trans Ultrason Ferroelectr Freq Control 2008; 55(6): 1316-27.[http://dx.doi.org/10.1109/TUFFC.2008.794] [PMID: 18599419]

[63] Berteau JP, Baron C, Pithioux M, Launay F, Chabrand P, Lasaygues P. *In vitro* ultrasonic and mechanic characterization of the modulus of elasticity of children cortical bone. Ultrasonics 2014; 54(5): 1270-6.[http://dx.doi.org/10.1016/j.ultras.2013.09.014] [PMID: 24112598]

[64] Eneh CT, Malo MK, Karjalainen JP, Liukkonen J, Töyräs J, Jurvelin JS. Effect of porosity, tissue density, and mechanical properties on radial sound speed in human cortical bone. Med Phys 2016; 43(5): 2030.[http://dx.doi.org/10.1118/1.4942808] [PMID: 27147315]

[65] Arendts FJ, Sigolotto C. Standard measurements, elasticity values and tensile strength behavior of the human mandible, a contribution to the biomechanics of the mandible--I. Biomed Tech (Berl) 1989; 34(10): 248-55.[http://dx.doi.org/10.1515/bmte.1989.34.10.248] [PMID: 2819111]

[66] Arendts FJ, Sigolotto C. Mechanical characteristics of the human mandible and study of *in vivo* behavior of compact bone tissue, a contribution to the description of biomechanics of the mandible--II. Biomed Tech (Berl) 1990; 35(6): 123-30.[http://dx.doi.org/10.1515/bmte.1990.35.6.123] [PMID: 2372566]

[67] O'Mahony AM, Williams JL, Katz JO, Spencer P. Anisotropic elastic properties of cancellous bone from a human edentulous mandible. Clin Oral Implants Res 2000; 11(5): 415-21.[http://dx.doi.org/10.1034/j.1600-0501.2000.011005415.x] [PMID: 11168233]

[68] Giesen EBW, Ding M, Dalstra M, van Eijden TMGJ. Mechanical properties of cancellous bone in the human mandibular condyle are anisotropic. J Biomech 2001; 34(6): 799-803 .[http://dx.doi.org/10.1016/S0021-9290(01)00030-6] [PMID: 11470118]

[69] Carter R. The elastic properties of the human mandible. Dissertation, New Orleans, Tulane University, 1989.

[70] Bacon GE, Bacon PJ, Griffiths RK. Orientation of apatite crystals in relation to muscle attachment in the mandible. J Biomech 1980; 13(8): 725-9.[http://dx.doi.org/10.1016/0021-9290(80)90358-9] [PMID: 7419538]

[71] Turner CH, Cowin SC, Rho JY, Ashman RB, Rice JC. The fabric dependence of the orthotropic elastic constants of cancellous bone. J Biomech 1990; 23(6): 549-561 .[http://dx.doi.org/10.1016/0021-9290(90)90048-8] [PMID: 2341418]

[72] Schwartz-Dabney CL, Dechow PC, Ashman RB. Elastic properties of human mandibular symphysis. J Dent Res 1991; 70: 518.

[73] Kingsmill VJ, Boyde A. Variation in the apparent density of human mandibular bone with age and dental status. J Anat 1998; 192(Pt 2): 233-44.[http://dx.doi.org/10.1046/j.1469-7580.1998.19220233.x] [PMID: 9643424]

[74] Kingsmill VJ, Boyde A. Mineralisation density of human mandibular bone: quantitative backscattered electron image analysis. J Anat 1998; 192(Pt 2): 245-256

.[http://dx.doi.org/10.1046/j.1469-7580.1998.19220245.x] [PMID: 9643425]

[75] Okeson JP. Fundamentals of occlusion and temporomandibular disorders. St Louis, The CV Mosby Co, 1985.

[76] OpenStax College. Anatomy and physiology. Houston: Rice University 2013.

[77] Berkovitz BKB, Holland GR, Moxham BJ. A colour atlas and textbook of oral anatomy. London, Wolfe Medical, 1978.

[78] Hildebrand GY. Studies in the masticatory movements of the lower jaw. Berlin, Walter De Gruyter, 1931.

[79] Adams SH II, Zander HA. Functional tooth contacts in lateral and centric occlusion. J Am Dent Assoc 1964; 69: 465-73.[http://dx.doi.org/10.14219/jada.archive.1964.0306] [PMID: 14198784]

[80] Glickman I, Pameijer JHN, Roeber FW, Brion MAM. Functional occlusion as revealed by miniaturized radio transmitters. Dent Clin North Am 1969; 13(3): 667-79.[PMID: 5255321]

[81] Suit SR, Gibbs CH, Benz ST. Study of gliding tooth contacts during mastication. J Periodontol 1976; 47(6): 331-4.[http://dx.doi.org/10.1902/jop.1976.47.6.331] [PMID: 1064720]

[82] Brekhus PH, Armstrong WD, Simon WJ. Stimulation of the muscles of mastication. J Dent Res 1941; 20: 87.[http://dx.doi.org/10.1177/00220345410200020801]

[83] Worner HK. Gnathodynamics: the measurements of biting force with a new design of gnathodynamometer. Dent J Aust 1939; 43: 381.

[84] Worner HK, Anderson MN. Biting force measurements in children. Aust Dent J 1944; 48: 1.

[85] Garner LD, Kotwal NS. Correlation study of incisive biting forces with age, sex, and anterior occlusion. J Dent Res 1973; 52(4): 698-702.[http://dx.doi.org/10.1177/00220345730520041001] [PMID: 4515849]

[86] Smith RJ. Mandibular biomechanics and temporomandibular joint function in primates. Am J Phys Anthropol 1978; 49(3): 341-9.[http://dx.doi.org/10.1002/ajpa.1330490307] [PMID: 103437]

[87] Robinson M. The temporomandibular joint; theory of reflex controlled nonlever action of the mandible. J Am Dent Assoc 1946; 33: 1260-71.[http://dx.doi.org/10.14219/jada.archive.1946.0176] [PMID: 21000178]

[88] Roberts D, Tattersall I. Skull form and the mechanics of mandibular elevation in mammals. Am Mus Novit 1974; 2356: 1-9.

[89] Grant PG. Biomechanical significance of the instantaneous center of rotation: the human temporomandibular joint. J Biomech 1973; 6(2): 109-113 .[http://dx.doi.org/10.1016/0021-9290(73)90080-8] [PMID: 4693143]

[90] Roberts D. The etiology of the temporomandibular joint dysfunction syndrome. Am J Orthod 1974; 66(5): 498-515.[http://dx.doi.org/10.1016/0002-9416(74)90111-0] [PMID: 4621248]

[91] Parrington FR. On the Cynodont genus Galesaurus, with a note on the functional significance of the changes in the evolution of the Theriodont skull. Ann Mag Nat Hist 1934; 13: 38-67.[http://dx.doi.org/10.1080/00222933408654791]

[92] Badoux DM. Statics of the mandible. Acta Morphol Neerl Scand 1966; 6(3): 251-6.[PMID: 6008210]

[93] Bock WJ. An approach to the functional analysis of bill shape. Auk 1966; 83: 10-51.[http://dx.doi.org/10.2307/4082976]

[94] Bock WJ, Kummer B. The avian mandible as a structural girder. J Biomech 1968; 1(2): 89-96.[http://dx.doi.org/10.1016/0021-9290(68)90011-0] [PMID: 16329296]

[95] Hylander WL. *In vivo* bone strain in the mandible of Galago crassicaudatus. Am J Phys Anthropol 1977; 46(2): 309-26.[http://dx.doi.org/10.1002/ajpa.1330460212] [PMID: 403774]

[96]   Stern JT Jr. Letter: Biomechanical significance of the instantaneous center of rotation: the human temporomandibular   joint.   J   Biomech   1974;   7(1):   109-110 .[http://dx.doi.org/10.1016/0021-9290(74)90075-X] [PMID: 4820645]

[97]   Hylander WL. The human mandible: lever or link? Am J Phys Anthropol 1975; 43(2): 227-42.[http://dx.doi.org/10.1002/ajpa.1330430209] [PMID: 1101706]

[98]   Hylander WL. Experimental analysis of temporomandibular joint reaction force in macaques. Am J Phys Anthropol 1979; 51(3): 433-56.[http://dx.doi.org/10.1002/ajpa.1330510317] [PMID: 532828]

[99]   Hylander WL. Stress and strain in the mandibular symphysis of primates: a test of competing hypotheses. Am J Phys Anthropol 1984; 64(1): 1-46.[http://dx.doi.org/10.1002/ajpa.1330640102] [PMID: 6731608]

[100]   Wilson GH. The anatomy and physics of the temporomandibular joint. J Nat Dent Assoc 1920; 7: 414-20.[http://dx.doi.org/10.14219/jada.archive.1920.0080]

[101]   Frank L. Muscular influence on occlusion as shown by x-rays of the condyle. Dent Dig 1950; 56(11): 484-8.[PMID: 14793022]

[102]   Gingerich PD. Functional significance of mandibular translation in vertebrate jaw mechanics. Postilla 1971; 152: 1-10.

[103]   Tattersall I. Cranial anatomy of archaeolmurinae (lemuroidea primates). Anthropol Pap Am Mus Nat Hist 1973; 52: 1-110.

[104]   Posselt U. Physiology of occlusion and rehabilitation. Oxford, Blackwell Scientific Publication, 1962.

[105]   Carlsoo S. Nervous co-ordination and mechanical function of the mandibular elevators. An EMG study of the activity, and an anatomic analysis of the mechanics of muscles. Acta Odont Scand 1952; 10: Suppl. 1-132.

[106]   Carlsoo S. Motor units and action potentials in masticatory muscles; an electromyographic study of the form and duration of the action potentials and an anatomic study of the size of the motor units. Acta Morphol Neerl Scand 1958; 2(1): 13-9.[PMID: 13594291]

[107]   Kawamura Y, Majima T, Kato I. Physiologic role of deep mechanoreceptor in temporomandibular joint capsule. J Osaka Univ Dent Sch 1967; 7: 63-76.[PMID: 5238355]

[108]   Lund P, Nishiyama T, Moller E. Postural activity in the muscles of mastication with the subject upright, inclined, and supine. Scand J Dent Res 1970; 78(5): 417-24.[PMID: 5275853]

[109]   Lehr RP, Blanton PL, Biggs NL. An electromyographic study of the mylohyoid muscle. Anat Rec 1971; 169(4): 651-60.[http://dx.doi.org/10.1002/ar.1091690405] [PMID: 5573345]

[110]   Messerman T, Reswick JB, Gibbs C. Investigation of functional mandibular movements. Dent Clin North Am 1969; 13(3): 629-42.[PMID: 5255319]

[111]   Moyers RE. An electromyographic analysis of certain muscles involved in temporomandibular movement. Am J Orthod 1950; 36(7): 481-515.[http://dx.doi.org/10.1016/0002-9416(50)90063-7] [PMID: 15425629]

[112]   Sicher H, Du Brul EL. Oral Anatomy. St Louis, CV Mosby, 1975.

[113]   Woelfel JB, Hickey JC, Stacy RW, Rinear LL. Electromyographic analysis of jaw movements. J Pros Dent 1960; 10: 688-98.[http://dx.doi.org/10.1016/0022-3913(60)90250-X]

[114]   Moller E. The chewing apparatus: an EMG study of the action of the muscles of mastication and its correlation to facial morphology. Acta Physiol Scand 1966; 69: Suppl. 280.

[115]   Amis AA, Dowson D, Wright V. Elbow joint force predictions for some strenuous isometric actions. J Biomech 1980; 13(9): 765-75.[http://dx.doi.org/10.1016/0021-9290(80)90238-9] [PMID: 7440591]

[116]   Throckmorton GS, Throckmorton LS. Quantitative calculations of temporomandibular joint reaction forces--I. The importance of the magnitude of the jaw muscle forces. J Biomech 1985; 18(6):

445-52.[http://dx.doi.org/10.1016/0021-9290(85)90279-9] [PMID: 3839795]

[117] Gysi A. Studies on the leverage problem of the mandible. Dent Dig 1921; 27: 74-84, 184-190, 203-208.

[118] Craddock FW. A review of Costen's syndrome. Br Dent J 1951; 91(8): 199-204.[PMID: 14886446]

[119] Roydhouse RH. The temporomandibular joint: upward force of the condyles on the cranium. J Am Dent Assoc 1955; 50(2): 166-72.[http://dx.doi.org/10.14219/jada.archive.1955.0043] [PMID: 13221384]

[120] Barbenel JC. The biomechanics of the temporomandibular joint: a theoretical study. J Biomech 1972; 5(3): 251-6.[http://dx.doi.org/10.1016/0021-9290(72)90039-5] [PMID: 4666528]

[121] Barbenel JC. The mechanics of the temporomandibular joint--a theoretical and electromyographical study. J Oral Rehabil 1974; 1(1): 19-27.[http://dx.doi.org/10.1111/j.1365-2842.1974.tb01262.x] [PMID: 4530054]

[122] Hylander WL. Incisal bite force direction in humans and the functional significance of mammalian mandibular translation. Am J Phys Anthropol 1978; 48(1): 1-7 .[http://dx.doi.org/10.1002/ajpa.1330480102] [PMID: 623224]

[123] Schumacher GH. Funktionelle Morphologie der Kinnmuskulatur. VEB. Jena, Gustav Fischer, 1961.

[124] Pruim GJ, de Jongh HJ, ten Bosch JJ. Forces acting on the mandible during bilateral static bite at different bite force levels. J Biomech 1980; 13(9): 755-763 .[http://dx.doi.org/10.1016/0021-9290(80)90237-7] [PMID: 7440590]

[125] Fick H. Handbuch der Anatomie und Mechanik der Gelenke. Jena, Gustav Fischer, 1904.

[126] Morris CB. The measurement of the strength of muscle relative to the cross section. Res Q 1948; 19(4): 295-303.[PMID: 18108557]

[127] Hettinger T. Physiology of strength. Illinois, Charles C Thomas, 1961.

[128] Ikai M, Fukunaga T. Calculation of muscle strength per unit cross-sectional area of human muscle by means of ultrasonic measurement. Int Z Angew Physiol 1968; 26(1): 26-32.[PMID: 5700894]

[129] Mainland D, Hiltz JE. Forces exerted on the human mandible by the muscles of mastication. J Dent Res 1934; 14: 107-24.[http://dx.doi.org/10.1177/00220345340140020101]

[130] Carlsoo S. An electromyographic study of the activity, and an anatomic analysis of the mechanics of the lateral pterygoid muscle. Acta Anat (Basel) 1956; 26(4): 339-351 .[http://dx.doi.org/10.1159/000141107] [PMID: 13338963]

[131] Pruim GJ, Ten Bosch JJ, de Jongh HJ. Jaw muscle EMG-activity and static loading of the mandible. J Biomech 1978; 11(8-9): 389-95.[http://dx.doi.org/10.1016/0021-9290(78)90073-8] [PMID: 711787]

[132] Osborn JW, Baragar FA. Predicted pattern of human muscle activity during clenching derived from a computer assisted model: symmetric vertical bite forces. J Biomech 1985; 18(8): 599-612.[http://dx.doi.org/10.1016/0021-9290(85)90014-4] [PMID: 4055814]

[133] Bock WJ. Mechanics of one- and two-joint muscles. Am Mus Novit 1986; 2319: 1-45.

[134] Pelosi G. The finite-element method, part I: R.L. Courant: historical corner. IEEE Antennas Propag Mag 2007; 49: 180-2.[http://dx.doi.org/10.1109/MAP.2007.376627]

[135] Courant RL. Variational methods for the solution of problems of equilibrium and vibrations. Bull Am Math Soc 1943; 49: 1-23.[http://dx.doi.org/10.1090/S0002-9904-1943-07818-4]

[136] Turner MJ, Clough RW, Martin HC, Topp LJ. Stiffness and deflection analysis of complex structures. J Aerosp Sci 1956; 23: 805-24.

[137] Turner MJ. The Direct Stiffness Method of Structural Analysis, Structural and Materials Panel Paper. AGARD Meeting. Aachen, Germany 1959.

[138] Turner MJ, Martin HC, Weikel RC. Further development and applications of the stiffness method. In: Fraeijs de Veubeke BM, Ed. AGARDograph 72: Matrix Methods of Structural Analysis. Oxford, Pergamon Press, 1964; pp. 203-66.

[139] Clough RW. The Finite Element Method in Plane Stress Analysis. Proceedings of the 2nd ASCE Conference on Electronic Computation Pittsburgh, USA. 1960.

[140] Clough RW. The finite element method - a personal view of its original formulation.From Finite Elements to the Troll Platform - the Ivar Holand 70th Anniversary Volume 1994; 89-100.

[141] Ciarlet PG. The finite element method for elliptic problems. Amsterdam,North-Holland Publishing, 1978.

[142] Brenner S, Scott RL. The mathematical theory of finite element methods. 2nd edition. New York, Springer, 2005.

[143] Zienkiewicz OC, Taylor RL. The finite element method 4th edition. London, McGraw-Hill Book Company (UK) Limited, 1991.

[144] Rho JY, Hobatho MC, Ashman RB. Relations of mechanical properties to density and CT numbers in human bone. Med Eng Phys 1995; 17(5): 347-55.[http://dx.doi.org/10.1016/1350-4533(95)97314-F] [PMID: 7670694]

[145] Hvid I, Bentzen SM, Linde F, Mosekilde L, Pongsoipetch B. X-ray quantitative computed tomography: the relations to physical properties of proximal tibial trabecular bone specimens. J Biomech 1989; 22(8-9): 837-44.[http://dx.doi.org/10.1016/0021-9290(89)90067-5] [PMID: 2613719]

[146] Peng L, Bai J, Zeng X, Zhou Y. Comparison of isotropic and orthotropic material property assignments on femoral finite element models under two loading conditions. Med Eng Phys 2006; 28(3): 227-33.[http://dx.doi.org/10.1016/j.medengphy.2005.06.003] [PMID: 16076560]

[147] Laz PJ, Stowe JQ, Baldwin MA, Petrella AJ, Rullkoetter PJ. Incorporating uncertainty in mechanical properties for finite element-based evaluation of bone mechanics. J Biomech 2007; 40(13): 2831-6.[http://dx.doi.org/10.1016/j.jbiomech.2007.03.013] [PMID: 17475268]

[148] Schwartz-Dabney CL, Dechow PC. Edentulation alters material properties of cortical bone in the human mandible. J Dent Res 2002; 81(9): 613-7.[http://dx.doi.org/10.1177/154405910208100907] [PMID: 12202642]

[149] Helgason B, Perilli E, Schileo E, Taddei F, Brynjólfsson S, Viceconti M. Mathematical relationships between bone density and mechanical properties: a literature review. Clin Biomech (Bristol, Avon) 2008; 23(2): 135-46.[http://dx.doi.org/10.1016/j.clinbiomech.2007.08.024] [PMID: 17931759]

[150] Carter DR, Hayes WC. Bone compressive strength: the influence of density and strain rate. Science 1976; 194(4270): 1174-6.[http://dx.doi.org/10.1126/science.996549] [PMID: 996549]

[151] Hernandez CJ, Beaupré GS, Keller TS, Carter DR. The influence of bone volume fraction and ash fraction on bone strength and modulus. Bone 2001; 29(1): 74-78 .[http://dx.doi.org/10.1016/S8756-3282(01)00467-7] [PMID: 11472894]

[152] Rice JC, Cowin SC, Bowman JA. On the dependence of the elasticity and strength of cancellous bone on apparent density. J Biomech 1988; 21(2): 155-168 .[http://dx.doi.org/10.1016/0021-9290(88)90008-5] [PMID: 3350829]

[153] Schaffler MB, Burr DB. Stiffness of compact bone: effects of porosity and density. J Biomech 1988; 21(1): 13-6.[http://dx.doi.org/10.1016/0021-9290(88)90186-8] [PMID: 3339022]

[154] Hodgskinson R, Currey JD. The effect of variation in structure on the Young's modulus of cancellous bone: a comparison of human and non-human material. Proc Inst Mech Eng H 1990; 204(2): 115-21.[http://dx.doi.org/10.1243/PIME_PROC_1990_204_240_02] [PMID: 2095142]

[155] Keller TS. Predicting the compressive mechanical behavior of bone. J Biomech 1994; 27(9): 1159-68.[http://dx.doi.org/10.1016/0021-9290(94)90056-6] [PMID: 7929465]

[156] Morgan EF, Bayraktar HH, Keaveny TM. Trabecular bone modulus-density relationships depend on anatomic site. J Biomech 2003; 36(7): 897-904.[http://dx.doi.org/10.1016/S0021-9290(03)00071-X] [PMID: 12757797]

[157] Poelert S, Valstar E, Weinans H, Zadpoor AA. Patient-specific finite element modeling of bones. Proc Inst Mech Eng H 2013; 227(4): 464-78.[http://dx.doi.org/10.1177/0954411912467884] [PMID: 23637222]

[158] Helgason B, Taddei F, Pálsson H, *et al.* A modified method for assigning material properties to FE models of bones. Med Eng Phys 2008; 30(4): 444-453 .[http://dx.doi.org/10.1016/j.medengphy.2007.05.006] [PMID: 17627862]

[159] Koseki M, Inou N, Maki K. Estimation of masticatory forces for patient-specific analysis of the human mandible.Modelling in Medicine and Biology VI 2005; 491-500 .[http://dx.doi.org/10.2495/BIO050471]

[160] Choi AH, Ben-Nissan B, Conway RC. Three-dimensional modelling and finite element analysis of the human mandible during clenching. Aust Dent J 2005; 50(1): 42-48 .[http://dx.doi.org/10.1111/j.1834-7819.2005.tb00084.x] [PMID: 15881305]

[161] Choi AH, Conway RC, Taraschi V, Ben-Nissan B. Biomechanics and functional distortion of the human mandible. J Investig Clin Dent 2015; 6(4): 241-51.[http://dx.doi.org/10.1111/jicd.12112] [PMID: 25044432]

[162] Bianco P, Riminucci M, Gronthos S, Robey PG. Bone marrow stromal stem cells: nature, biology, and potential applications. Stem Cells 2001; 19(3): 180-92.[http://dx.doi.org/10.1634/stemcells.19-3-180] [PMID: 11359943]

[163] Hadjidakis DJ, Androulakis II. Bone remodeling. Ann N Y Acad Sci 2006; 1092: 385-396 .[http://dx.doi.org/10.1196/annals.1365.035] [PMID: 17308163]

[164] Teitelbaum SL. Bone resorption by osteoclasts. Science 2000; 289(5484): 1504-1508 .[http://dx.doi.org/10.1126/science.289.5484.1504] [PMID: 10968780]

[165] Choi AH, Conway RC, Ben-Nissan B. Finite-element modeling and analysis in nanomedicine and dentistry. Nanomedicine (Lond) 2014; 9(11): 1681-95.[http://dx.doi.org/10.2217/nnm.14.75] [PMID: 25321169]

[166] Byrne DP, Lacroix D, Prendergast PJ. Simulation of fracture healing in the tibia: mechanoregulation of cell activity using a lattice modeling approach. J Orthop Res 2011; 29(10): 1496-503.[http://dx.doi.org/10.1002/jor.21362] [PMID: 21462249]

[167] Isaksson H. Recent advances in mechanobiological modeling of bone regeneration. Mech Res Commun 2012; 42: 22-31.[http://dx.doi.org/10.1016/j.mechrescom.2011.11.006]

[168] Grivas KN, Vavva MG, Sellountos EJ, Polyzos D, Fotiadis DI. A meshless Local Boundary Integral Equation (LBIE) method for cell proliferation predictions in bone healing. Conf Proc IEEE Eng Med Biol Soc 2013; 2013: 2676-9.[PMID: 24110278]

[169] Alierta JA, Pérez MA, García-Aznar JM. An interface finite element model can be used to predict healing outcome of bone fractures. J Mech Behav Biomed Mater 2014; 29: 328-38.[http://dx.doi.org/10.1016/j.jmbbm.2013.09.023] [PMID: 24145150]

[170] García-Aznar JM, Kuiper JH, Gómez-Benito MJ, Doblaré M, Richardson JB. Computational simulation of fracture healing: influence of interfragmentary movement on the callus growth. J Biomech 2007; 40(7): 1467-76.[http://dx.doi.org/10.1016/j.jbiomech.2006.06.013] [PMID: 16930609]

[171] Comiskey D, MacDonald BJ, McCartney WT, Synnott K, O'Byrne J. Predicting the external formation of callus tissues in oblique bone fractures: idealised and clinical case studies. Biomech Model Mechanobiol 2013; 12(6): 1277-82.[http://dx.doi.org/10.1007/s10237-012-0468-6] [PMID: 23306603]

[172] Kimsal J, Baack B, Candelaria L, Khraishi T, Lovald S. Biomechanical analysis of mandibular angle

fractures. J Oral Maxillofac Surg 2011; 69(12): 3010-4.[http://dx.doi.org/10.1016/j.joms.2010.12.042] [PMID: 21496988]

[173] Vajgel A, Camargo IB, Willmersdorf RB, de Melo TM, Laureano Filho JR, Vasconcellos RJ. Comparative finite element analysis of the biomechanical stability of 2.0 fixation plates in atrophic mandibular fractures. J Oral Maxillofac Surg 2013; 71(2): 335-342 .[http://dx.doi.org/10.1016/j.joms.2012.09.019] [PMID: 23351762]

[174] Joshi U, Kurakar M. Comparison of stability of fracture segments in mandible fracture treated with different designs of mini-plates using FEM analysis. J Maxillofac Oral Surg 2014; 13(3): 310-9.[http://dx.doi.org/10.1007/s12663-013-0510-y] [PMID: 25018606]

[175] Albougha S, Darwich K, Darwich MA, Albogha MH. Assessment of sagittal split ramus osteotomy rigid internal fixation techniques using a finite element method. Int J Oral Maxillofac Surg 2015; 44(7): 823-9.[http://dx.doi.org/10.1016/j.ijom.2015.02.006] [PMID: 25766461]

[176] Murakami K, Yamamoto K, Sugiura T, Kawakami M, Horita S, Kirita T. Biomechanical analysis of poly-L-lactic acid and titanium plates fixated for mandibular symphyseal fracture with a conservatively treated unilateral condylar fracture using the three-dimensional finite element method. Dent Traumatol 2015; 31(5): 396-402.[http://dx.doi.org/10.1111/edt.12179] [PMID: 25976121]

[177] Darwich MA, Albogha MH, Abdelmajeed A, Darwich K. Assessment of the biomechanical performance of 5 plating techniques in fixation of mandibular subcondylar fracture using finite element analysis. J Oral Maxillofac Surg 2016; 74(4): 794.e1-794.e8 .[http://dx.doi.org/10.1016/j.joms.2015.11.021] [PMID: 26706490]

[178] Pituru TS, Bucur A, Gudas C, Pituru SM, Marius Dinca O. New miniplate for osteosynthesis of mandibular angle fractures designed to improve formation of new bone. J Craniomaxillofac Surg 2016; 44(4): 500-5.[http://dx.doi.org/10.1016/j.jcms.2016.01.002] [PMID: 26888464]

[179] Tanaka E, Yamamoto S, Nishida T, Aoki Y. A mathematical model of bone remodeling under overload and its application to evaluation of bone resorption around dental implants. Acta Bioeng Biomech 1999; 1: 117-21.

[180] Huiskes R, Weinans H, Grootenboer HJ, Dalstra M, Fudala B, Slooff TJ. Adaptive bone-remodeling theory applied to prosthetic-design analysis. J Biomech 1987; 20(11-12): 1135-1150 .[http://dx.doi.org/10.1016/0021-9290(87)90030-3] [PMID: 3429459]

[181] Huiskes R. Validation of adaptive bone-remodeling simulation models. Stud Health Technol Inform 1997; 40: 33-48.[PMID: 10168881]

[182] Carter DR. Mechanical loading histories and cortical bone remodeling. Calcif Tissue Int 1984; 36 (Suppl. 1): S19-24.[http://dx.doi.org/10.1007/BF02406129] [PMID: 6430518]

[183] Mellal A, Wiskott HW, Botsis J, Scherrer SS, Belser UC. Stimulating effect of implant loading on surrounding bone. Comparison of three numerical models and validation by *in vivo* data. Clin Oral Implants Res 2004; 15(2): 239-48.[http://dx.doi.org/10.1111/j.1600-0501.2004.01000.x] [PMID: 15008937]

[184] Lin CL, Lin YH, Chang SH. Multi-factorial analysis of variables influencing the bone loss of an implant placed in the maxilla: prediction using FEA and SED bone remodeling algorithm. J Biomech 2010; 43(4): 644-51.[http://dx.doi.org/10.1016/j.jbiomech.2009.10.030] [PMID: 19939391]

[185] Galbusera F, Taschieri S, Tsesis I, Francetti L, Del Fabbro M. Finite element simulation of implant placement following extraction of a single tooth. J Appl Biomater Funct Mater 2014; 12(2): 84-9.[http://dx.doi.org/10.5301/JABFM.5000178] [PMID: 24425378]

[186] Lee WT, Koak JY, Lim YJ, Kim SK, Kwon HB, Kim MJ. Stress shielding and fatigue limits of poly-ether-ether-ketone dental implants. J Biomed Mater Res B Appl Biomater 2012; 100(4): 1044-52.[http://dx.doi.org/10.1002/jbm.b.32669] [PMID: 22331553]

[187] Wang C, Li Q, McClean C, Fan Y. Numerical simulation of dental bone remodeling induced by implant-supported fixed partial denture with or without cantilever extension. Int J Numer Methods

Biomed Eng 2013; 29(10): 1134-47.[http://dx.doi.org/10.1002/cnm.2579] [PMID: 23873599]

[188] Rungsiyakull C, Chen J, Rungsiyakull P, Li W, Swain M, Li Q. Bone's responses to different designs of implant-supported fixed partial dentures. Biomech Model Mechanobiol 2015; 14(2): 403-11.[http://dx.doi.org/10.1007/s10237-014-0612-6] [PMID: 25209424]

[189] Suenaga H, Chen J, Yamaguchi K, *et al.* Mechanobiological bone reaction quantified by positron emission tomography. J Dent Res 2015; 94(5): 738-44.[http://dx.doi.org/10.1177/0022034515573271] [PMID: 25710952]

[190] Carter DR. Mechanical loading history and skeletal biology. J Biomech 1987; 20(11-12): 1095-109.[http://dx.doi.org/10.1016/0021-9290(87)90027-3] [PMID: 3323201]

[191] Beaupré GS, Orr TE, Carter DR. An approach for time-dependent bone modeling and remodeling-theoretical development. J Orthop Res 1990; 8(5): 651-61.[http://dx.doi.org/10.1002/jor.1100080506] [PMID: 2388105]

[192] Eser A, Tonuk E, Akca K, Cehreli MC. Predicting time-dependent remodeling of bone around immediately loaded dental implants with different designs. Med Eng Phys 2010; 32(1): 22-31.[http://dx.doi.org/10.1016/j.medengphy.2009.10.004] [PMID: 19884034]

[193] Sotto-Maior BS, Mercuri EG, Senna PM, Assis NM, Francischone CE, Del Bel Cury AA. Evaluation of bone remodeling around single dental implants of different lengths: a mechanobiological numerical simulation and validation using clinical data. Comput Methods Biomech Biomed Engin 2016; 19(7): 699-706.[http://dx.doi.org/10.1080/10255842.2015.1052418] [PMID: 26249362]

[194] Eser A, Tonuk E, Akca K, Dard MM, Cehreli MC. Predicting bone remodeling around tissue- and bone-level dental implants used in reduced bone width. J Biomech 2013; 46(13): 2250-7.[http://dx.doi.org/10.1016/j.jbiomech.2013.06.025] [PMID: 23876712]

[195] Weinans H, Huiskes R, Grootenboer HJ. The behavior of adaptive bone-remodeling simulation models. J Biomech 1992; 25(12): 1425-41.[http://dx.doi.org/10.1016/0021-9290(92)90056-7] [PMID: 1491020]

[196] Lin D, Li Q, Li W, Duckmanton N, Swain M. Mandibular bone remodeling induced by dental implant. J Biomech 2010; 43(2): 287-93.[http://dx.doi.org/10.1016/j.jbiomech.2009.08.024] [PMID: 19815211]

[197] Wang C, Wang L, Liu X, Fan Y. Numerical simulation of the remodelling process of trabecular architecture around dental implants. Comput Methods Biomech Biomed Engin 2014; 17(3): 286-95.[http://dx.doi.org/10.1080/10255842.2012.681646] [PMID: 22571498]

[198] McNamara LM, Prendergast PJ. Bone remodelling algorithms incorporating both strain and microdamage stimuli. J Biomech 2007; 40(6): 1381-1391 .[http://dx.doi.org/10.1016/j.jbiomech.2006.05.007] [PMID: 16930610]

[199] Carter DR, Hayes WC, Schurman DJ. Fatigue life of compact bone--II. Effects of microstructure and density. J Biomech 1976; 9(4): 211-8.[http://dx.doi.org/10.1016/0021-9290(76)90006-3] [PMID: 1262355]

[200] Chou HY, Romanos G, Müftü A, Müftü S. Peri-implant bone remodeling around an extraction socket: predictions of bone maintenance by finite element method. Int J Oral Maxillofac Implants 2012; 27(4): e39-48.[PMID: 22848899]

[201] Moreo P, García-Aznar JM, Doblaré M. Bone ingrowth on the surface of endosseous implants. Part 1: Mathematical model. J Theor Biol 2009; 260(1): 1-12.[http://dx.doi.org/10.1016/j.jtbi.2008.07.040] [PMID: 18762197]

[202] Vanegas-Acosta JC, Landinez P NS, Garzón-Alvarado DA, Casale R MC. A finite element method approach for the mechanobiological modeling of the osseointegration of a dental implant. Comput Methods Programs Biomed 2011; 101(3): 297-314.[http://dx.doi.org/10.1016/j.cmpb.2010.11.007] [PMID: 21183241]

[203] Ben-Nissan B, Choi AH, Cordingley RC. Alumina ceramics. In: Kokubo T, Ed. Bioceramics and their

clinical applications. England, Woodhead Publishing, 2008; pp. 233-42.

[204] Thompson ID, Hench LL. Mechanical properties of bioactive glasses, glass-ceramics and composites. Proc Inst Mech Eng H 1998; 212(2): 127-36.[http://dx.doi.org/10.1243/0954411981533908] [PMID: 9612004]

[205] Clupper DC, Gough JE, Embanga PM, Notingher I, Hench LL, Hall MM. Bioactive evaluation of 45S5 bioactive glass fibres and preliminary study of human osteoblast attachment. J Mater Sci Mater Med 2004; 15(7): 803-8.[http://dx.doi.org/10.1023/B:JMSM.0000032821.32577.fc] [PMID: 15387416]

[206] Clupper DC, Hench LL, Mecholsky JJ. Strength and toughness of tape cast bioactive glass 45S5 following heat treatment. J Eur Ceram Soc 2004; 24: 2929-2934 .[http://dx.doi.org/10.1016/S0955-2219(03)00363-7]

[207] Willmann G. Ceramics for total hip replacement--what a surgeon should know. Orthopedics 1998; 21(2): 173-7.[PMID: 9507269]

[208] Hench LL. Bioactive ceramics. In: Ducheyne P, Lemons JE, Eds. Bioceramics: materials characteristics vs. in vivo behavior. New York, Annual of the New York Academy of Science, 1988; pp. 54-71.[http://dx.doi.org/10.1111/j.1749-6632.1988.tb38500.x]

[209] Duret F, Blouin JL, Duret B. CAD-CAM in dentistry. J Am Dent Assoc 1988; 117(6): 715-20.[http://dx.doi.org/10.14219/jada.archive.1988.0096] [PMID: 3058771]

[210] Zarina R, Jaini JL, Raj RS. Evolution of the Software and Hardware in CAD/CAM Systems used in Dentistry. Int J Prev Clin Dent Res 2017; 4: 1-8.[http://dx.doi.org/10.5005/jp-journals-10052-0127]

[211] Strub JR, Rekow ED, Witkowski S. Computer-aided design and fabrication of dental restorations: current systems and future possibilities. J Am Dent Assoc 2006; 137(9): 1289-96.[http://dx.doi.org/10.14219/jada.archive.2006.0389] [PMID: 16946436]

[212] Choi AH, Ben-Nissan B, Conway RC. Finite Element Analysis (FEA) in Dentistry. In: Matinlinna JP, Ed. Handbook of Oral Biomaterials. Singapore, Pan Stanford Publishing, 2012; pp. 535-76.

[213] Ferrage L, Bertrand G, Lenormand P, Grossin D, Ben-Nissan B. A review of the additive manufacturing (3DP) of bioceramics: alumina, zirconia (PSZ) and hydroxyapatite. J Aust Ceram Soc 2017; 53: 11-20.[http://dx.doi.org/10.1007/s41779-016-0003-9]

[214] de Groot K, Geesink R, Klein CPAT, Serekian P. Plasma sprayed coatings of hydroxylapatite. J Biomed Mater Res 1987; 21(12): 1375-81.[http://dx.doi.org/10.1002/jbm.820211203] [PMID: 3429472]

[215] Hench LL. Bioceramics: from concept to clinic. J Am Ceram Soc 1991; 74: 1487-1510 .[http://dx.doi.org/10.1111/j.1151-2916.1991.tb07132.x]

[216] Choi AH, Ben-Nissan B, Matinlinna JP, Conway RC. Current perspectives: calcium phosphate nanocoatings and nanocomposite coatings in dentistry. J Dent Res 2013; 92(10): 853-859 .[http://dx.doi.org/10.1177/0022034513497754] [PMID: 23857642]

[217] LeGeros RZ. Biodegradation and bioresorption of calcium phosphate ceramics. Clin Mater 1993; 14(1): 65-88.[http://dx.doi.org/10.1016/0267-6605(93)90049-D] [PMID: 10171998]

[218] Ben-Nissan B, Choi AH. Sol-gel production of bioactive nanocoatings for medical applications. Part 1: an introduction. Nanomedicine (Lond) 2006; 1(3): 311-9.[http://dx.doi.org/10.2217/17435889.1.3.311] [PMID: 17716161]

[219] Choi AH, Ben-Nissan B. Sol-gel production of bioactive nanocoatings for medical applications. Part II: current research and development. Nanomedicine (Lond) 2007; 2(1): 51-61 .[http://dx.doi.org/10.2217/17435889.2.1.51] [PMID: 17716190]

[220] LeGeros RZ. Properties of osteoconductive biomaterials: calcium phosphates. Clin Orthop Relat Res 2002; (395): 81-98.[http://dx.doi.org/10.1097/00003086-200202000-00009] [PMID: 11937868]

[221] Ben-Nissan B, Milev A, Vago R. Morphology of sol-gel derived nano-coated coralline hydroxyapatite. Biomaterials 2004; 25(20): 4971-5.[http://dx.doi.org/10.1016/j.biomaterials.2004.02.006] [PMID: 15109858]

[222] Hu J, Russell JJ, Ben-Nissan B, Vago R. Production and analysis of hydroxyapatite from Australian corals via hydrothermal process. J Mater Sci Lett 2001; 20: 85-87 .[http://dx.doi.org/10.1023/A:1006735319725]

[223] Ben-Nissan B, Milev A, Vago R, Conway M, Diwan A. Sol-gel derived nano-coated coralline hydroxyapatite for load bearing applications. Key Eng Mater 2004; 254-256: 301-304 .[http://dx.doi.org/10.4028/www.scientific.net/KEM.254-256.301]

[224] Depprich R, Zipprich H, Ommerborn M, *et al.* Osseointegration of zirconia implants: an SEM observation of the bone-implant interface. Head Face Med 2008; 4: 25 .[http://dx.doi.org/10.1186/1746-160X-4-25] [PMID: 18990214]

[225] Choi AH, Matinlinna JP, Ben-Nissan B. Finite element stress analysis of Ti-6Al-4V and partially stabilized zirconia dental implant during clenching. Acta Odontol Scand 2012; 70(5): 353-61.[http://dx.doi.org/10.3109/00016357.2011.600723] [PMID: 21815837]

[226] Choi AH, Matinlinna J, Ben-Nissan B. Effects of micromovement on the changes in stress distribution of partially stabilized zirconia (PS-ZrO$_2$) dental implants and bridge during clenching: a three-dimensional finite element analysis. Acta Odontol Scand 2013; 71(1): 72-81 .[http://dx.doi.org/10.3109/00016357.2011.654242] [PMID: 22364339]

[227] Giordano R, Sabrosa CE. Zirconia: material background and clinical application. Compend Contin Educ Dent 2010; 31(9): 710-5.[PMID: 21197939]

[228] Chevalier J, Gremillard L. Zirconia ceramics.Bioceramics and their clinical applications 2008; 243-65.[http://dx.doi.org/10.1533/9781845694227.2.243]

[229] Manicone PF, Rossi Iommetti P, Raffaelli L. An overview of zirconia ceramics: basic properties and clinical applications. J Dent 2007; 35(11): 819-26.[http://dx.doi.org/10.1016/j.jdent.2007.07.008] [PMID: 17825465]

[230] Clarke IC, Manaka M, Green DD, *et al.* Current status of zirconia used in total hip implants. J Bone Joint Surg Am 2003; 85-A (Suppl. 4): 73-84.[http://dx.doi.org/10.2106/00004623-200300004-00009] [PMID: 14652396]

[231] Garvie RC, Hannink RH, Pascoe RT. Ceramic steel? Nature 1975; 258: 703-704 .[http://dx.doi.org/10.1038/258703a0]

[232] Yoshimura M, Noma T, Kawabata K, Somiya S. Role of H$_2$O on the degradation process of Y-TZP. J Mater Sci Lett 1987; 6: 465.[http://dx.doi.org/10.1007/BF01756800]

[233] Piconi C, Maccauro G. Zirconia as a ceramic biomaterial. Biomaterials 1999; 20(1): 1-25.[http://dx.doi.org/10.1016/S0142-9612(98)00010-6] [PMID: 9916767]

[234] Willmann G. The color of bioceramics. Key Eng Mater 2003; 240-242: 785-788 .[http://dx.doi.org/10.4028/www.scientific.net/KEM.240-242.785]

[235] Huckstep RL, Sherry E. Replacement of the proximal humerus in primary bone tumours. Aust N Z J Surg 1996; 66(2): 97-100.[http://dx.doi.org/10.1111/j.1445-2197.1996.tb01121.x] [PMID: 8602824]

[236] Oonishi H, Takayaka Y, Clarke IC, Jung H. Comparative wear studies of 28-mm ceramic and stainless steel total hip joints over a two to seven year period. J Long Term Eff Med Implants 1992; 2: 37-47.

[237] Oonishi H, Clarke IC, Good V, *et al.* Needs of bioceramics to longevity of total joint arthroplasty. Key Eng Mater 2003; 240-242: 735-54.[http://dx.doi.org/10.4028/www.scientific.net/KEM.240-242.735]

[238] Sedel L. Evolution of alumina-on-alumina implants: a review. Clin Orthop Relat Res 2000; (379): 48-54.[http://dx.doi.org/10.1097/00003086-200010000-00008] [PMID: 11039792]

[239] Insley GM, Turner I, Fisher J, Streicher RM. *In vitro* testing and validation of zirconia toughened

alumina. In: Proceedings of the 7th Biolox® symposium. Stuttgart, Germany, 2007; pp. 26-31.

[240] Hench LL, West JK. Biological applications of bioactive glasses. Life Chem Rep 1996; 13: 187-241.

[241] Marrelli M, Falisi G, Apicella A, *et al.* Behaviour of dental pulp stem cells on different types of innovative mesoporous and nanoporous silicon scaffolds with different functionalizations of the surfaces. J Biol Regul Homeost Agents 2015; 29(4): 991-7.[PMID: 26753666]

[242] Ben-Nissan B, Choi AH, Macha I. Advances in bioglass and glass ceramics for biomedical applications. In: Li Q, Mai YW, Eds. Biomaterials for implants and scaffolds. Germany, Springer Series in Biomaterials Science and Engineering (SSBSE), 2017; pp. 133-61.[http://dx.doi.org/10.1007/978-3-662-53574-5_5]

[243] Hench LL, Splinter RJ, Allen WC, Greenlee TK. Bonding mechanisms at the interface of ceramic prosthetic materials. J Biomed Mater Res Symp 1972; 2: 117-41.

[244] Vrouwenvelder WCA, Groot CG, de Groot K. Histological and biochemical evaluation of osteoblasts cultured on bioactive glass, hydroxylapatite, titanium alloy, and stainless steel. J Biomed Mater Res 1993; 27(4): 465-75.[http://dx.doi.org/10.1002/jbm.820270407] [PMID: 8385144]

[245] Andersson OH, Kangasniemi I. Calcium phosphate formation at the surface of bioactive glass *in vitro*. J Biomed Mater Res 1991; 25(8): 1019-30.[http://dx.doi.org/10.1002/jbm.820250808] [PMID: 1918106]

[246] Li P, Yang Q, Zhang F, Kokubo T. The effect of residual glassy phase in a bioactive glass-ceramic on the formation of its surface apatite layer *in vitro*. J Mater Sci Mater Med 1992; 3: 452-6.[http://dx.doi.org/10.1007/BF00701242]

[247] Kokubo T, Shigematsu M, Nagashima Y, *et al.* Apatite-wollastonite containing glass-ceramic for prosthetic application. Bull Inst Chem Res 1982; 60: 260-8.

[248] Andersson ÖH. Glass transition temperature of glasses in the SiO_2-Na_2O-CaO-P_2O_5-Al_2O_3-B_2O_3 system. J Mater Sci Mater Med 1992; 3: 326-8.[http://dx.doi.org/10.1007/BF00705363]

[249] Peitl Filho O, LaTorre GP, Hench LL. Effect of crystallization on apatite-layer formation of bioactive glass 45S5. J Biomed Mater Res 1996; 30(4): 509-514 .[http://dx.doi.org/10.1002/(SICI)1097-4636(199604)30:4<509::AID-JBM9>3.0.CO;2-T] [PMID: 8847359]

[250] Hayakawa S, Tsuru K, Ohtsuki C. Mechanism of apatite formation on a sodium silicate glass in a simulated body fluid. J Am Ceram Soc 1999; 82: 2155-2160 .[http://dx.doi.org/10.1111/j.1151-2916.1999.tb02056.x]

[251] Arstila H, Vedel E, Hupa L, Ylänen HO, Hupa M. Measuring the devitrification of bioactive glasses. Key Eng Mater 2004; 254-256: 67-70.[http://dx.doi.org/10.4028/www.scientific.net/KEM.254-256.67]

[252] Ylänen HO, Helminen T, Helminen A, Rantakokko J, Karlsson KH, Aro HT. Porous bioactive glass matrix in reconstruction of articular osteochondral defects. Ann Chir Gynaecol 1999; 88(3): 237-45.[PMID: 10532567]

[253] Fröberg L, Hupa L, Hupa M. Porous bioactive glasses with controlled mechanical strength. Key Eng Mater 2004; 254-256: 973-6.[http://dx.doi.org/10.4028/www.scientific.net/KEM.254-256.973]

[254] Niki M, Ito G, Matsuda T, Ogino M. Comparative push-out data of bioactive and non-bioactive materials of similar rugosity.Bone-material interface 1991; 350-356 .[http://dx.doi.org/10.3138/9781442671508-035]

[255] Wilson J, Pigott GH, Schoen FJ, Hench LL. Toxicology and biocompatibility of bioglasses. J Biomed Mater Res 1981; 15(6): 805-17.[http://dx.doi.org/10.1002/jbm.820150605] [PMID: 7309763]

[256] Fujiu T, Ogino M. Difference of bond bonding behavior among surface active glasses and sintered apatite. J Biomed Mater Res 1984; 18(7): 845-59.[http://dx.doi.org/10.1002/jbm.820180714] [PMID: 6544783]

[257] Andersson ÖH, Karlsson KH, Kangasniemi K. Calcium-phosphate formation at the surface of bioactive glass *in vivo*. J Non-Cryst Solids 1990; 119: 290-296 .[http://dx.doi.org/10.1016/0022-3093(90)90301-2]

[258] LeGeros RZ, LeGeros JP. Dense hydroxyapatite. In: Hench LL, Wilson J, Eds. An introduction to bioceramics, Vol. 1. Singapore, World Scientific, 1993; pp. 139-80.[http://dx.doi.org/10.1142/9789814317351_0009]

[259] Lai W, Ducheyne P, Garino J. Removal pathway of silicon released from bioactive glass granules *in vivo*. In: LeGeros RZ, LeGeros JP Eds. Bioceramics. New York, World Scientific, 1998; pp. 383-6.

[260] Oonishi H, Hench LL, Wilson J, *et al.* Quantitative comparison of bone growth behavior in granules of Bioglass, A-W glass-ceramic, and hydroxyapatite. J Biomed Mater Res 2000; 51(1): 37-46.[http://dx.doi.org/10.1002/(SICI)1097-4636(200007)51:1<37::AID-JBM6>3.0.CO;2-T] [PMID: 10813743]

[261] Hench LL. Glass and genes: a forecast to future. Glastech Ber Glass Sci Technol 1997; 70: 439-52.

[262] Hench LL. Bioceramics. J Am Ceram Soc 1998; 81: 1705-1727 .[http://dx.doi.org/10.1111/j.1151-2916.1998.tb02540.x]

[263] Strnad Z. Role of the glass phase in bioactive glass-ceramics. Biomaterials 1992; 13(5): 317-21.[http://dx.doi.org/10.1016/0142-9612(92)90056-T] [PMID: 1600033]

[264] Karlsson KH, Ylänen HO. Porous bone implants. In: Vincenzini P, Ed. Materials in clinical applications, advances in science and technology 28. Florence, 9th Cimtec-World Forum on New Materials, 1998.

[265] Serra J, González P, Liste S, *et al.* Influence of the non-bridging oxygen groups on the bioactivity of silicate glasses. J Mater Sci Mater Med 2002; 13(12): 1221-1225 .[http://dx.doi.org/10.1023/A:1021174912802] [PMID: 15348669]

[266] Serra J, González P, Liste S, *et al.* FTIR and XPS studies of bioactive silica based glasses. J Non-Cryst Solids 2003; 332: 20-7.[http://dx.doi.org/10.1016/j.jnoncrysol.2003.09.013]

[267] Ducheyne P, Brown S, Blumenthal N, *et al.* Bioactive glasses, aluminum oxide, and titanium. Ion transport phenomena and surface analysis. Ann N Y Acad Sci 1988; 523: 257-61.[http://dx.doi.org/10.1111/j.1749-6632.1988.tb38517.x] [PMID: 3382125]

[268] Li R, Clark AE, Hench LL. An investigation of bioactive glass powders by sol-gel processing. J Appl Biomater 1991; 2(4): 231-9.[http://dx.doi.org/10.1002/jab.770020403] [PMID: 10171144]

[269] Boccaccini AR, Erol M, Stark WJ, Mohn D, Hong Z, Mano JF. Polymer/bioactive glass nanocomposites for biomedical applications: A review. Compos Sci Technol 2010; 70: 1764-76.[http://dx.doi.org/10.1016/j.compscitech.2010.06.002]

[270] Stark WJ, Mädler L, Maciejewski M, Pratsinis SE, Baiker A. Flame synthesis of nanocrystalline ceria-zirconia: effect of carrier liquid. Chem Commun (Camb) 2003; 5(5): 588-9.[http://dx.doi.org/10.1039/b211831a] [PMID: 12669838]

[271] Madler L, Stark WJ, Pratsinis SE. Flame-made ceria nanoparticles. J Mater Res 2002; 17: 1356-62.[http://dx.doi.org/10.1557/JMR.2002.0202]

[272] Athanassiou EK, Grass RN, Stark WJ. Chemical aerosol engineering as a novel tool for material science: from oxides to salt and metal nanoparticles. Aerosol Sci Technol 2010; 44: 161-72.[http://dx.doi.org/10.1080/02786820903449665]

[273] Vollenweider M, Brunner TJ, Knecht S, *et al.* Remineralization of human dentin using ultrafine bioactive glass particles. Acta Biomater 2007; 3(6): 936-943 .[http://dx.doi.org/10.1016/j.actbio.2007.04.003] [PMID: 17560183]

[274] Mohn D, Zehnder M, Imfeld T, Stark WJ. Radio-opaque nanosized bioactive glass for potential root canal application: evaluation of radiopacity, bioactivity and alkaline capacity. Int Endod J 2010; 43(3):

210-7.[http://dx.doi.org/10.1111/j.1365-2591.2009.01660.x] [PMID: 20158532]

[275] Quinteroa F, Dieste O, Pou J, Lusquiños F, Riveiro A. On the conditions to produce micro- and nanofibers by laser spinning. J Phys D Appl Phys 2009; 42: 1-10.

[276] Quintero F, Pou J, Comesana R, *et al.* Laser spinning of bioactive glass nanofibers. Adv Funct Mater 2009; 19: 3084-90.[http://dx.doi.org/10.1002/adfm.200801922]

[277] Quintero F, Pou J, Lusquiños F, Riveiro A. Experimental analysis of the production of micro- and nanofibers by laser spinning. Appl Surf Sci 2007; 254: 1042-1047 .[http://dx.doi.org/10.1016/j.apsusc.2007.07.190]

[278] Arriagada FJ, Osseo-Asare K. Synthesis of nanosize silica in a nonionic water-in-oil microemulsion: effects of the water/surfactant molar ratio and ammonia concentration. J Colloid Interface Sci 1999; 211(2): 210-20.[http://dx.doi.org/10.1006/jcis.1998.5985] [PMID: 10049537]

[279] Singh S, Bhardwaj P, Singh V, Aggarwal S, Mandal UK. Synthesis of nanocrystalline calcium phosphate in microemulsion--effect of nature of surfactants. J Colloid Interface Sci 2008; 319(1): 322-9.[http://dx.doi.org/10.1016/j.jcis.2007.09.059] [PMID: 18083184]

[280] Karagiozov C, Momchilova D. Synthesis of nano-sized particles from metal carbonates by the method of reversed mycelles. Chem Eng Process 2005; 44: 115-119 .[http://dx.doi.org/10.1016/j.cep.2004.05.004]

[281] Sun Y, Guo G, Tao D, Wang ZH. Reverse microemulsion-directed synthesis of hydroxyapatite nanoparticles under hydrothermal conditions. J Phys Chem Solids 2007; 68: 373-7.[http://dx.doi.org/10.1016/j.jpcs.2006.11.026]

[282] Lim GK, Wang J, Ng SC, Gan LM. Processing of fine hydroxyapatite powders via an inverse microemulsion route. Mater Lett 1996; 28: 431-6.[http://dx.doi.org/10.1016/0167-577X(96)00095-X]

[283] Lim GK, Wang J, Ng SC, Gan LM. Formation of Nanocrystalline hydroxyapatite in nonionic surfactant emulsions. Langmuir 1999; 15: 7472-7.[http://dx.doi.org/10.1021/la981659+]

[284] Hench LL, West JK. The sol-gel process. Chem Rev 1990; 90: 33-72.[http://dx.doi.org/10.1021/cr00099a003]

[285] Greenspan DC, Zhong JP, Chen XF, LaTorre GP. The evaluation of degradability of melt and sol-gel derived Bioglass® *in-vitro*. Bioceramics 1997; 10: 391-4.

[286] Jie Q, Lin K, Zhong J, *et al.* Preparation of macroporous sol-gel bioglass using PVA particles as pore former. J Sol-Gel Sci Technol 2004; 30: 49-61 .[http://dx.doi.org/10.1023/B:JSST.0000028196.09929.a3]

[287] Saboori A, Rabiee M, Moztarzadeh F, Sheikhi M, Tahriri M, Karimi M. Synthesis, characterization and in vitro bioactivity of sol-gel-derived SiO2-CaO-P2O5-MgO bioglass. Mat Sci Eng C-Bio 2009; S 29: 335-340.

[288] Chen QZ, Thouas GA. Fabrication and characterization of sol-gel derived 45S5 Bioglass®-ceramic scaffolds. Acta Biomater 2011; 7(10): 3616-26.[http://dx.doi.org/10.1016/j.actbio.2011.06.005] [PMID: 21689791]

[289] Cacciotti I, Lombardi M, Bianco A, Ravaglioli A, Montanaro L. Sol-gel derived 45S5 bioglass: synthesis, microstructural evolution and thermal behaviour. J Mater Sci Mater Med 2012; 23(8): 1849-66.[http://dx.doi.org/10.1007/s10856-012-4667-6] [PMID: 22580755]

[290] Sakka S. Glasses and glass-ceramics from gels. J Non-Cryst Solids 1985; 73: 651.[http://dx.doi.org/10.1016/0022-3093(85)90385-0]

[291] Pereira MM, Hench LL. Mechanisms of hydroxyapatite formation on porous gel-silica substrates. J Sol-Gel Sci Technol 1996; 7: 59-68.[http://dx.doi.org/10.1007/BF00401884]

[292] Hench LL, Greenspan D. Interactions between bioactive glass and collagen: a review and new perspectives. J Aust Ceram Soc 2013; 49: 1-40.

[293] Ylänen HO. Bone ingrowth into porous bodies made by sintering bioactive glass microspheres, Dissertation, Åbo Akademi University, 2000.

[294] Wilson J, Yli-Urpo A, Happonen RP. Bioactive glasses: clinical applications. In: Hench LL, Wilson J, Eds. An introduction to bioceramics. Singapore, World Scientific, 1993; pp. 63-73.[http://dx.doi.org/10.1142/9789814317351_0004]

[295] Stoor P, Söderling E, Salonen JI. Antibacterial effects of a bioactive glass paste on oral microorganisms. Acta Odontol Scand 1998; 56(3): 161-165 .[http://dx.doi.org/10.1080/000163598422901] [PMID: 9688225]

[296] Stoor P, Söderling E, Grenman R. Interactions between the bioactive glass S53P4 and the atrophic rhinitis-associated microorganism klebsiella ozaenae. J Biomed Mater Res 1999; 48(6): 869-74.[http://dx.doi.org/10.1002/(SICI)1097-4636(1999)48:6<869::AID-JBM16>3.0.CO;2-6] [PMID: 10556853]

[297] Stoor P, Pulkkinen J, Grénman R. Bioactive glass S53P4 in the filling of cavities in the mastoid cell area in surgery for chronic otitis media. Ann Otol Rhinol Laryngol 2010; 119(6): 377-82.[http://dx.doi.org/10.1177/000348941011900603] [PMID: 20583735]

[298] Suominen E, Kinnunen J. Bioactive glass granules and plates in the reconstruction of defects of the facial bones. Scand J Plast Reconstr Surg Hand Surg 1996; 30(4): 281-9.[http://dx.doi.org/10.3109/02844319609056406] [PMID: 8976023]

[299] Kinnunen I, Aitasalo K, Pöllönen M, Varpula M. Reconstruction of orbital floor fractures using bioactive glass. J Craniomaxillofac Surg 2000; 28(4): 229-234 .[http://dx.doi.org/10.1054/jcms.2000.0140] [PMID: 11110155]

[300] Stanley HR, Hall MB, Clark AE, King CJ III, Hench LL, Berte JJ. Using 45S5 bioglass cones as endosseous ridge maintenance implants to prevent alveolar ridge resorption: a 5-year evaluation. Int J Oral Maxillofac Implants 1997; 12(1): 95-105.[PMID: 9048461]

[301] Hench LL. Bioceramics, a clinical success. Am Ceram Soc Bull 1998; 77: 67-74.

[302] Croteau S, Rauch F, Silvestri A, Hamdy RC. Bone morphogenetic proteins in orthopedics: from basic science to clinical practice. Orthopedics 1999; 22(7): 686-95.[PMID: 10418866]

[303] Harakas NK. Demineralized bone-matrix-induced osteogenesis. Clin Orthop Relat Res 1984; (188): 239-51.[PMID: 6380863]

[304] Zhang N, Nichols HL, Taylor S, Wen X. Fabrication of nanocrystalline hydroxyapatite doped degradable composite hollow fiber for guided and biomimetic bone tissue engineering. Mater Sci Eng 2007; 27: 599-606.[http://dx.doi.org/10.1016/j.msec.2006.05.024]

[305] Peroglio M, Gremillard L, Chevalier J, Chazeau L, Gauthier C, Hamaide T. Toughening of bio-ceramics scaffolds by polymer coating. J Eur Ceram Soc 2007; 27: 2679-2685 .[http://dx.doi.org/10.1016/j.jeurceramsoc.2006.10.016]

[306] Albee FH, Morrison HF. Studies in bone growth: Triple CaP as a stimulus to osteogenesis. Ann Surg 1920; 71(1): 32-9.[http://dx.doi.org/10.1097/00000658-192001000-00006] [PMID: 17864220]

[307] Hulbert SF, Young FA, Mathews RS, Klawitter JJ, Talbert CD, Stelling FH. Potential of ceramic materials as permanently implantable skeletal prostheses. J Biomed Mater Res 1970; 4(3): 433-56.[http://dx.doi.org/10.1002/jbm.820040309] [PMID: 5469185]

[308] Choi AH, Ben-Nissan B. Calcium Phosphate Nanocomposites for Biomedical and Dental Applications: Recent Developments. In: Thakur VK, Thakur MK, Kessler MR, Eds. V.K. Thakur, M.K. Thakur, and M.R. Kessler, Vol. 8. Massachusetts, Scrivener Publishing, 2017; pp. 423-50.[http://dx.doi.org/10.1002/9781119441632.ch163]

[309] Murugan R, Ramakrishna S. Development of nanocomposites for bone grafting. Compos Sci Technol 2005; 65: 2385-406.[http://dx.doi.org/10.1016/j.compscitech.2005.07.022]

[310] Oliveira JM, Rodrigues MT, Silva SS, *et al.* Novel hydroxyapatite/chitosan bilayered scaffold for osteochondral tissue-engineering applications: Scaffold design and its performance when seeded with goat bone marrow stromal cells. Biomaterials 2006; 27(36): 6123-6137 .[http://dx.doi.org/10.1016/j.biomaterials.2006.07.034] [PMID: 16945410]

[311] Wahl DA, Czernuszka JT. Collagen-hydroxyapatite composites for hard tissue repair. Eur Cell Mater 2006; 11: 43-56.[http://dx.doi.org/10.22203/eCM.v011a06] [PMID: 16568401]

[312] Hild N, Fuhrer R, Mohn D, *et al.* Nanocomposites of high-density polyethylene with amorphous calcium phosphate: *in vitro* biomineralization and cytocompatibility of human mesenchymal stem cells. Biomed Mater 2012; 7(5): 054103.[http://dx.doi.org/10.1088/1748-6041/7/5/054103] [PMID: 22972023]

[313] TenHuisen KS, Martin RI, Klimkiewicz M, Brown PW. Formation and properties of a synthetic bone composite: hydroxyapatite-collagen. J Biomed Mater Res 1995; 29(7): 803-810 .[http://dx.doi.org/10.1002/jbm.820290704] [PMID: 7593018]

[314] Scabbia A, Trombelli L. A comparative study on the use of a HA/collagen/chondroitin sulphate biomaterial (Biostite) and a bovine-derived HA xenograft (Bio-Oss) in the treatment of deep intra-osseous defects. J Clin Periodontol 2004; 31(5): 348-355 .[http://dx.doi.org/10.1111/j.1600-051X.2004.00483.x] [PMID: 15086616]

[315] Ebrahimi M, Pripatnanont P, Monmaturapoj N, Suttapreyasri S. Fabrication and characterization of novel nano hydroxyapatite/β-tricalcium phosphate scaffolds in three different composition ratios. J Biomed Mater Res A 2012; 100(9): 2260-8.[PMID: 22499354]

[316] Daculsi G, Passuti N, Martin S, Deudon C, Legeros RZ, Raher S. Macroporous calcium phosphate ceramic for long bone surgery in humans and dogs. Clinical and histological study. J Biomed Mater Res 1990; 24(3): 379-96.[http://dx.doi.org/10.1002/jbm.820240309] [PMID: 2318901]

[317] Nery EB, LeGeros RZ, Lynch KL, Lee K. Tissue response to biphasic calcium phosphate ceramic with different ratios of HA/β TCP in periodontal osseous defects. J Periodontol 1992; 63(9): 729-35.[http://dx.doi.org/10.1902/jop.1992.63.9.729] [PMID: 1335498]

[318] LeGeros RZ, Lin S, Rohanizadeh R, Mijares D, LeGeros JP. Biphasic calcium phosphate bioceramics: preparation, properties and applications. J Mater Sci Mater Med 2003; 14(3): 201-209 .[http://dx.doi.org/10.1023/A:1022872421333] [PMID: 15348465]

[319] Azevedo MC, Reis RL, Claase MB, Grijpma DW, Feijen J. Development and properties of polycaprolactone/hydroxyapatite composite biomaterials. J Mater Sci Mater Med 2003; 14(2): 103-7.[http://dx.doi.org/10.1023/A:1022051326282] [PMID: 15348480]

[320] Lee JH, Rim NG, Jung HS, Shin H. Control of osteogenic differentiation and mineralization of human mesenchymal stem cells on composite nanofibers containing poly[lactic-co-(glycolic acid)] and hydroxyapatite. Macromol Biosci 2010; 10(2): 173-82.[http://dx.doi.org/10.1002/mabi.200900169] [PMID: 19685498]

[321] Lock J, Nguyen TY, Liu H. Nanophase hydroxyapatite and poly(lactide-co-glycolide) composites promote human mesenchymal stem cell adhesion and osteogenic differentiation *in vitro*. J Mater Sci Mater Med 2012; 23(10): 2543-52.[http://dx.doi.org/10.1007/s10856-012-4709-0] [PMID: 22772475]

[322] Buschmann J, Härter L, Gao S, *et al.* Tissue engineered bone grafts based on biomimetic nanocomposite PLGA/amorphous calcium phosphate scaffold and human adipose-derived stem cells. Injury 2012; 43(10): 1689-97.[http://dx.doi.org/10.1016/j.injury.2012.06.004] [PMID: 22769980]

[323] Guo J, Meng Z, Chen G, *et al.* Restoration of critical-size defects in the rabbit mandible using porous nanohydroxyapatite-polyamide scaffolds. Tissue Eng Part A 2012; 18(11-12): 1239-1252 .[http://dx.doi.org/10.1089/ten.tea.2011.0503] [PMID: 22320360]

[324] Huang D, Zuo Y, Zou Q, *et al.* Reinforced nanohydroxyapatite/polyamide66 scaffolds by chitosan coating for bone tissue engineering. J Biomed Mater Res B Appl Biomater 2012; 100(1): 51-57 .[http://dx.doi.org/10.1002/jbm.b.31921] [PMID: 21953937]

[325] Yang X, Yang F, Walboomers XF, Bian Z, Fan M, Jansen JA. The performance of dental pulp stem cells on nanofibrous PCL/gelatin/nHA scaffolds. J Biomed Mater Res A 2010; 93(1): 247-57.[PMID: 19557787]

[326] Fletcher J, Walsh D, Fowler CE, Mann S. Electrospun mats of PVP/ACP nanofibres for remineralization of enamel tooth surfaces. CrystEngComm 2011; 13: 3692-3697 .[http://dx.doi.org/10.1039/c0ce00806k]

[327] Huang JS, Liu KM, Chen CC, *et al.* Liposomes-coated hydroxyapatite and tricalcium phosphate implanted in the mandibular bony defect of miniature swine. Kaohsiung J Med Sci 1997; 13(4): 213-28.[PMID: 9177083]

[328] Ono I, Yamashita T, Jin HY, *et al.* Combination of porous hydroxyapatite and cationic liposomes as a vector for BMP-2 gene therapy. Biomaterials 2004; 25(19): 4709-4718 .[http://dx.doi.org/10.1016/j.biomaterials.2003.11.038] [PMID: 15120517]

[329] Merwin GE. Review of bioactive materials for otologic and maxillofacial applications. In: Yamamuro T, Hench LL, Wilson J, Eds. Handbook of bioactive ceramics, Vol. 1. Florida, CRC Press, 1990; pp. 323-8.

[330] Cai YR, Zhou L. Effect of thermal treatment on the microstructure and mechanical properties of gel-derived bioglasses. Mater Chem Phys 2005; 94: 283-287 .[http://dx.doi.org/10.1016/j.matchemphys.2005.04.050]

[331] Hench LL. The story of Bioglass. J Mater Sci Mater Med 2006; 17(11): 967-78.[http://dx.doi.org/10.1007/s10856-006-0432-z] [PMID: 17122907]

[332] Jones JR, Ehrenfried LM, Hench LL. Optimising bioactive glass scaffolds for bone tissue engineering. Biomaterials 2006; 27(7): 964-73.[http://dx.doi.org/10.1016/j.biomaterials.2005.07.017] [PMID: 16102812]

[333] Heikkilä JT, Aho AJ, Yli-Urpo A, Andersson OH, Aho HJ, Happonen RP. Bioactive glass versus hydroxylapatite in reconstruction of osteochondral defects in the rabbit. Acta Orthop Scand 1993; 64(6): 678-82.[http://dx.doi.org/10.3109/17453679308994597] [PMID: 8291417]

[334] Suominen E, Aho AJ, Vedel E, Kangasniemi I, Uusipaikka E, Yli-Urpo A. Subchondral bone and cartilage repair with bioactive glasses, hydroxyapatite, and hydroxyapatite-glass composite. J Biomed Mater Res 1996; 32(4): 543-551 .[http://dx.doi.org/10.1002/(SICI)1097-4636(199612)32:4<543::AID-JBM7>3.0.CO;2-R] [PMID: 8953144]

[335] Aho AJ, Tirri T, Kukkonen J, *et al.* Injectable bioactive glass/biodegradable polymer composite for bone and cartilage reconstruction: concept and experimental outcome with thermoplastic composites of poly(epsilon-caprolactone-co-D,L-lactide) and bioactive glass S53P4. J Mater Sci Mater Med 2004; 15(10): 1165-73.[http://dx.doi.org/10.1023/B:JMSM.0000046401.50406.9b] [PMID: 15516880]

[336] Schepers E, de Clercq M, Ducheyne P, Kempeneers R. Bioactive glass particulate material as a filler for bone lesions. J Oral Rehabil 1991; 18(5): 439-452 .[http://dx.doi.org/10.1111/j.1365-2842.1991.tb01689.x] [PMID: 1666125]

[337] Gatti AM, Zaffe D, Gatti AM, Zaffe D. Long-term behaviour of active glasses in sheep mandibular bone. Biomaterials 1991; 12(3): 345-50.[http://dx.doi.org/10.1016/0142-9612(91)90044-B] [PMID: 1854903]

[338] García AJ, Ducheyne P. Numerical analysis of extracellular fluid flow and chemical species transport around and within porous bioactive glass. J Biomed Mater Res 1994; 28(8): 947-960 .[http://dx.doi.org/10.1002/jbm.820280814] [PMID: 7983093]

[339] Gatti AM, Valdrè G, Tombesi A. Importance of microanalysis in understanding mechanism of transformation in active glassy biomaterials. J Biomed Mater Res 1996; 31(4): 475-480 .[http://dx.doi.org/10.1002/(SICI)1097-4636(199608)31:4<475::AID-JBM6>3.0.CO;2-I] [PMID: 8836843]

[340] Heikkilä JT, Aho HJ, Yli-Urpo A, Happonen RP, Aho AJ. Bone formation in rabbit cancellous bone defects filled with bioactive glass granules. Acta Orthop Scand 1995; 66(5): 463-467 .[http://dx.doi.org/10.3109/17453679508995588] [PMID: 7484131]

[341] Oonishi H, Hench LL, Wilson J, *et al.* Comparative bone growth behavior in granules of bioceramic materials of various sizes. J Biomed Mater Res 1999; 44(1): 31-43 .[http://dx.doi.org/10.1002/(SICI)1097-4636(199901)44:1<31::AID-JBM4>3.0.CO;2-9] [PMID: 10397902]

[342] Virolainen P, Heikkilä J, Yli-Urpo A, Vuorio E, Aro HT. Histomorphometric and molecular biologic comparison of bioactive glass granules and autogenous bone grafts in augmentation of bone defect healing. J Biomed Mater Res 1997; 35(1): 9-17 .[http://dx.doi.org/10.1002/(SICI)1097-4636(199704)35:1<9::AID-JBM2>3.0.CO;2-S] [PMID: 9104694]

[343] Inchingolo F, Marrelli M, Annibali S, *et al.* Influence of endodontic treatment on systemic oxidative stress. Int J Med Sci 2013; 11(1): 1-6.[http://dx.doi.org/10.7150/ijms.6663] [PMID: 24396280]

[344] Marrelli M, Gentile S, Palmieri F, Paduano F, Tatullo M. Correlation between Surgeon's experience, surgery complexity and the alteration of stress related physiological parameters. PLoS One 2014; 9(11): e112444.[http://dx.doi.org/10.1371/journal.pone.0112444] [PMID: 25379944]

[345] Ben-Nissan B, Choi AH, Bendavid A. Mechanical properties of inorganic biomedical thin films and their corresponding testing methods. Surf Coat Tech 2013; 233: 39-48 .[http://dx.doi.org/10.1016/j.surfcoat.2012.11.020]

[346] Eger M, Sterer N, Liron T, Kohavi D, Gabet Y. Scaling of titanium implants entrains inflammation-induced osteolysis. Sci Rep 2017; 7: 39612.[http://dx.doi.org/10.1038/srep39612] [PMID: 28059080]

[347] Kirk PB, Filiaggi MJ, Sodhi RN, Pilliar RM. Evaluating sol-gel ceramic thin films for metal implant applications: III. *In vitro* aging of sol-gel-derived zirconia films on Ti-6Al-4V. J Biomed Mater Res 1999; 48(4): 424-433 .[http://dx.doi.org/10.1002/(SICI)1097-4636(1999)48:4<424::AID-JBM5>3.0.CO;2-1] [PMID: 10421683]

[348] Ducheyne P, Radin S, Heughebaert M, Heughebaert JC. Calcium phosphate ceramic coatings on porous titanium: effect of structure and composition on electrophoretic deposition, vacuum sintering and *in vitro* dissolution. Biomaterials 1990; 11(4): 244-254 .[http://dx.doi.org/10.1016/0142-9612(90)90005-B] [PMID: 2383619]

[349] Kokubo T, Kim HM, Kawashita M, Nakamura T. Novel ceramics for biomedical applications. J Aust Ceram Soc 2000; 36: 37-46.

[350] Colling EW. The physical metallurgy of titanium alloys.Cleveland, American Society for Metals, 1984.

[351] Gross KA, Saber-Samandari S. Revealing mechanical properties of a suspension plasma sprayed coating with nanoindentation. Surf Coat Tech 2009; 203: 2995-2999 .[http://dx.doi.org/10.1016/j.surfcoat.2009.03.007]

[352] Lin CK, Berndt CC. Measurement and analysis of adhesion strength for thermally sprayed coatings. J Thermal Spray Technol 1994; 3: 75-104.[http://dx.doi.org/10.1007/BF02649003]

[353] Ebelmen J. Untersuchungen über die verbindung der borsaure und kieselsaure mit aether. Ann Chim Phys Ser 1849; 57: 319-55.

[354] Geffcken W, Berger E. Änderung des reflexionsvermögens optischer gläser. German Patent 736411, 1939.

[355] Roy DM, Roy R. An experimental study of the formation and properties of synthetic serpentines and related layer silicates. Am Mineral 1954; 39: 957-75.

[356] Floch HG, Belleville PF, Priotton JJ, Pegon PM, Dijonneau CS, Guerain J. Sol-gel optical coatings for lasers. Int Am Ceram Soc Bull 1995; 74: 60-3.

[357] Percy MJ, Bartlett JR, Spiccia L, West BO, Woolfrey JL. The influence of b-diketones on hydrolysis and particle growth from zirconium (IV) N-propoxide in n-propanol. J Sol-Gel Sci Technol 2000; 19: 315-9.[http://dx.doi.org/10.1023/A:1008781515324]

[358] Harris MT, Byers CH, Brunson RR. A study of solvent effects on the synthesis of pure component and composite ceramic powders by metal alkoxide hydrolysis. Proc MRS 1988; 121: 287-292 .[http://dx.doi.org/10.1557/PROC-121-287]

[359] de Kambilly H, Klein LC. Effect of methanol concentration on lithium aluminosilicates. J Non-Cryst Solids 1989; 109: 69-78.[http://dx.doi.org/10.1016/0022-3093(89)90444-4]

[360] Anderson P, Klein LC. Shrinkage of lithium aluminosilicate gels during drying. J Non-Cryst Solids 1987; 93: 415-22.[http://dx.doi.org/10.1016/S0022-3093(87)80186-2]

[361] Pettit RB, Ashley CS, Reed ST, Brinker CJ. Antireflective films from the sol-gel process. In: Klein LC, Ed. Sol-Gel Technology for Thin Films, Fibers, Performs, Electronics, and Specialty Shapes. Park Ridge, Noyes Publishing, 1988; pp. 80-109.

[362] Sakka S, Kamiya K, Makita K, Tamamoto Y. Formation of sheets and coating films from alkoxide solutions. J Non-Cryst Solids 1984; 63: 223-35.[http://dx.doi.org/10.1016/0022-3093(84)90401-0]

[363] Strawbridge I, James PF. Thin silica films prepared by dip coating. J Non-Cryst Solids 1986; 82: 366-72.[http://dx.doi.org/10.1016/0022-3093(86)90153-5]

[364] Dislich H. Thin films from the sol-gel process. In: Klein LC, Ed. Sol-Gel Technology for Thin Films, Fibers, Performs, Electronics, and Specialty Shapes. Park Ridge, Noyes Publishing, 1988; pp. 55-77.

[365] Aksakal B, Hanyaloglu C. Bioceramic dip-coating on Ti-6Al-4V and 316L SS implant materials. J Mater Sci Mater Med 2008; 19(5): 2097-104.[http://dx.doi.org/10.1007/s10856-007-3304-2] [PMID: 17968501]

[366] Hu MS, Evans AG. The cracking and decohesion of thin films on ductile substrates. Acta Metall 1989; 37: 917-25.[http://dx.doi.org/10.1016/0001-6160(89)90018-7]

[367] Masuda Y, Matubara K, Sakka S. Synthesis of hydroxyapatite from metal alkoxides through sol-gel technique. J Ceram Soc Jpn 1990; 98: 1255-66.[http://dx.doi.org/10.2109/jcersj.98.1255]

[368] Chai CS, Gross KA, Ben-Nissan B. Critical ageing of hydroxyapatite sol-gel solutions. Biomaterials 1998; 19(24): 2291-6.[http://dx.doi.org/10.1016/S0142-9612(98)90138-7] [PMID: 9884042]

[369] Milev A, Kannangara GSK, Ben-Nissan B. Morphological stability of plate-like carbonate hydroxyapatite. Mater Lett 2003; 57: 1960-5.[http://dx.doi.org/10.1016/S0167-577X(02)01112-6]

[370] Scriven LE. Physics and application of dip coating and spin coating. Proc MRS 1988; 121: 717-29.[http://dx.doi.org/10.1557/PROC-121-717]

[371] Turner CW. Sol-gel process-Principles and applications. Ceram Bull 1991; 70: 1487-90.

[372] Lee JW, Won CW, Chun BS, Sohn HY. Dip-coating of alumina films by the sol-gel method. J Mater Res 1993; 8: 3151-7.[http://dx.doi.org/10.1557/JMR.1993.3151]

[373] Paterson MJ, Paterson PJK, Ben-Nissan B. The dependence of structural and mechanical properties on film thickness in sol-gel zirconia films. J Mater Res 1998; 13: 388 .[http://dx.doi.org/10.1557/JMR.1998.0051]

[374] Ducheyne P, Hench LL, Kagan A II, Martens M, Bursens A, Mulier JC. Effect of hydroxyapatite impregnation on skeletal bonding of porous coated implants. J Biomed Mater Res 1980; 14(3): 225-37.[http://dx.doi.org/10.1002/jbm.820140305] [PMID: 7364787]

[375] Li H, Khor KA, Cheang P. Adhesive and bending failure of thermal sprayed hydroxyapatite coatings: effect of nanostructures at interface and crack propagation phenomenon during bending. Eng Fract Mech 2007; 74: 1894-903.[http://dx.doi.org/10.1016/j.engfracmech.2006.06.001]

[376] Kim HW, Koh YH, Li LH, Lee S, Kim HE. Hydroxyapatite coating on titanium substrate with titania

buffer layer processed by sol-gel method. Biomaterials 2004; 25(13): 2533-2538 .[http://dx.doi.org/10.1016/j.biomaterials.2003.09.041] [PMID: 14751738]

[377] Lee HU, Jeong YS, Park SY, Jeong SY, Kim HG, Cho CR. Surface properties and cell response of fluoridated hydroxyapatite/TiO$_2$ coated on Ti substrate. Curr Appl Phys 2009; 9: 528-533 .[http://dx.doi.org/10.1016/j.cap.2008.03.020]

[378] Roest R, Latella BA, Heness G, Ben-Nissan B. Adhesion of sol-gel derived hydroxyapatite nanocoatings on anodized pure titanium and titanium (Ti6Al4V) alloy substrates. Surf Coat Tech 2011; 205: 3520-9.[http://dx.doi.org/10.1016/j.surfcoat.2010.12.030]

[379] Balakrishnan A, Lee BC, Kim TN, Panigrahi BB. Hydroxyapatite coatings on NaOH treated Ti-6A-
-4V alloy using sol-gel precursor. Mater Sci Technol 2007; 23: 1005-1007 .[http://dx.doi.org/10.1179/174328407X157380]

[380] Negroiu G, Piticescu RM, Chitanu GC, Mihailescu IN, Zdrentu L, Miroiu M. Biocompatibility evaluation of a novel hydroxyapatite-polymer coating for medical implants (in vitro tests). J Mater Sci Mater Med 2008; 19(4): 1537-44.[http://dx.doi.org/10.1007/s10856-007-3300-6] [PMID: 17990076]

[381] Gonzalez-McQuire R, Green DW, Partridge KA, Oreffo ROC, Mann S, Davis SA. Coating of human mesenchymal cells in 3D culture with bioinorganic nanoparticles promotes osteoblastic differentiation and gene transfection. Adv Mater 2007; 19: 2236-40.[http://dx.doi.org/10.1002/adma.200602770]

[382] Tatullo M, Marrelli M, Paduano F. The regenerative medicine in oral and maxillofacial surgery: the most important innovations in the clinical application of mesenchymal stem cells. Int J Med Sci 2015; 12(1): 72-7.[http://dx.doi.org/10.7150/ijms.10706] [PMID: 25552921]

[383] Tatullo M, Codispoti B, Pacifici A, *et al.* Potential use of human periapical cyst-mesenchymal stem cells (hPCy-MSCs) as a novel stem cell source for regenerative medicine applications. Front Cell Dev Biol 2017; 5: 103.[http://dx.doi.org/10.3389/fcell.2017.00103] [PMID: 29259970]

[384] Marrelli M, Paduano F, Tatullo M. Cells isolated from human periapical cysts express mesenchymal stem cell-like properties. Int J Biol Sci 2013; 9(10): 1070-8.[http://dx.doi.org/10.7150/ijbs.6662] [PMID: 24250252]

[385] Tatullo M, Falisi G, Amantea M, Rastelli C, Paduano F, Marrelli M. Dental pulp stem cells and human periapical cyst mesenchymal stem cells in bone tissue regeneration: comparison of basal and osteogenic differentiated gene expression of a newly discovered mesenchymal stem cell lineage. J Biol Regul Homeost Agents 2015; 29(3): 713-8.[PMID: 26403412]

[386] Fan Y, Duan K, Wang R. A composite coating by electrolysis-induced collagen self-assembly and calcium phosphate mineralization. Biomaterials 2005; 26(14): 1623-1632 .[http://dx.doi.org/10.1016/j.biomaterials.2004.06.019] [PMID: 15576136]

[387] Otsuka M, Nakagawa H, Ito A, Higuchi WI. Effect of geometrical structure on drug release rate of a three-dimensionally perforated porous apatite/collagen composite cement. J Pharm Sci 2010; 99(1): 286-92.[http://dx.doi.org/10.1002/jps.21835] [PMID: 19821491]

[388] de Jonge LT, Leeuwenburgh SC, van den Beucken JJ, *et al.* The osteogenic effect of electrosprayed nanoscale collagen/calcium phosphate coatings on titanium. Biomaterials 2010; 31(9): 2461-9.[http://dx.doi.org/10.1016/j.biomaterials.2009.11.114] [PMID: 20022365]

[389] Uezono M, Takakuda K, Kikuchi M, Suzuki S, Moriyama K. Hydroxyapatite/collagen nanocomposite-coated titanium rod for achieving rapid osseointegration onto bone surface. J Biomed Mater Res B Appl Biomater 2013; 101(6): 1031-8.[http://dx.doi.org/10.1002/jbm.b.32913] [PMID: 23554303]

[390] Chen D, Zhao M, Mundy GR. Bone morphogenetic proteins. Growth Factors 2004; 22(4): 233-241 .[http://dx.doi.org/10.1080/08977190412331279890] [PMID: 15621726]

[391] Urist MR. Bone: formation by autoinduction. Science 1965; 150(3698): 893-899 .[http://dx.doi.org/10.1126/science.150.3698.893] [PMID: 5319761]

[392] Wozney JM, Rosen V, Celeste AJ, *et al.* Novel regulators of bone formation: molecular clones and activities. Science 1988; 242(4885): 1528-34.[http://dx.doi.org/10.1126/science.3201241] [PMID: 3201241]

[393] Luyten FP, Cunningham NS, Ma S, *et al.* Purification and partial amino acid sequence of osteogenin, a protein initiating bone differentiation. J Biol Chem 1989; 264(23): 13377-80.[PMID: 2547759]

[394] Wozney JM. The bone morphogenetic protein family and osteogenesis. Mol Reprod Dev 1992; 32(2): 160-7.[http://dx.doi.org/10.1002/mrd.1080320212] [PMID: 1637554]

[395] Urist MR, DeLange RJ, Finerman GA. Bone cell differentiation and growth factors. Science 1983; 220(4598): 680-6.[http://dx.doi.org/10.1126/science.6403986] [PMID: 6403986]

[396] Urist MR, Nilsson O, Rasmussen J, *et al.* Bone regeneration under the influence of a bone morphogenetic protein (BMP) beta tricalcium phosphate (TCP) composite in skull trephine defects in dogs. Clin Orthop Relat Res 1987; (214): 295-304.[PMID: 3791755]

[397] Toriumi DM, Kotler HS, Luxenberg DP, Holtrop ME, Wang EA. Mandibular reconstruction with a recombinant bone-inducing factor. Functional, histologic, and biomechanical evaluation. Arch Otolaryngol Head Neck Surg 1991; 117(10): 1101-1112 .[http://dx.doi.org/10.1001/archotol.1991.01870220049009] [PMID: 1910694]

[398] Nevins M, Kirker-Head C, Nevins M, Wozney JA, Palmer R, Graham D. Bone formation in the goat maxillary sinus induced by absorbable collagen sponge implants impregnated with recombinant human bone morphogenetic protein-2. Int J Periodontics Restorative Dent 1996; 16(1): 8-19.[PMID: 8631615]

[399] Howell TH, Fiorellini J, Jones A, *et al.* A feasibility study evaluating rhBMP-2/absorbable collagen sponge device for local alveolar ridge preservation or augmentation. Int J Periodontics Restorative Dent 1997; 17(2): 124-39.[PMID: 9497707]

[400] Boyne PJ, Marx RE, Nevins M, *et al.* A feasibility study evaluating rhBMP-2/absorbable collagen sponge for maxillary sinus floor augmentation. Int J Periodontics Restorative Dent 1997; 17(1): 11-25.[PMID: 10332250]

[401] Fiorellini JP, Buser D, Riley E, Howell TH. Effect on bone healing of bone morphogenetic protein placed in combination with endosseous implants: a pilot study in beagle dogs. Int J Periodontics Restorative Dent 2001; 21(1): 41-7.[PMID: 11829034]

[402] Hanisch O, Tatakis DN, Boskovic MM, Rohrer MD, Wikesjö UM. Bone formation and reosseointegration in peri-implantitis defects following surgical implantation of rhBMP-2. Int J Oral Maxillofac Implants 1997; 12(5): 604-10.[PMID: 9337020]

[403] Sigurdsson TJ, Fu E, Tatakis DN, Rohrer MD, Wikesjö UM. Bone morphogenetic protein-2 for peri-implant bone regeneration and osseointegration. Clin Oral Implants Res 1997; 8(5): 367-74.[http://dx.doi.org/10.1034/j.1600-0501.1997.080503.x] [PMID: 9612141]

[404] Cochran DL, Schenk R, Buser D, Wozney JM, Jones AA. Recombinant human bone morphogenetic protein-2 stimulation of bone formation around endosseous dental implants. J Periodontol 1999; 70(2): 139-50.[http://dx.doi.org/10.1902/jop.1999.70.2.139] [PMID: 10102551]

[405] Tatakis DN, Koh A, Jin L, Wozney JM, Rohrer MD, Wikesjö UM. Peri-implant bone regeneration using recombinant human bone morphogenetic protein-2 in a canine model: a dose-response study. J Periodontal Res 2002; 37(2): 93-100.[http://dx.doi.org/10.1034/j.1600-0765.2002.00021.x] [PMID: 12009189]

[406] Rey C, Combes C, Drouet C, Sfihi H, Barroug A. Physico-chemical properties of nanocrystalline apatites: implications for biominerals and biomaterials. Mater Sci Eng C -. BIOS 2007; 27: 198-205.

[407] Liu Y, de Groot K, Hunziker EB. BMP-2 liberated from biomimetic implant coatings induces and sustains direct ossification in an ectopic rat model. Bone 2005; 36(5): 745-757 .[http://dx.doi.org/10.1016/j.bone.2005.02.005] [PMID: 15814303]

[408]   Liu Y, Enggist L, Kuffer AF, Buser D, Hunziker EB. The influence of BMP-2 and its mode of delivery on the osteoconductivity of implant surfaces during the early phase of osseointegration. Biomaterials 2007; 28(16): 2677-86.[http://dx.doi.org/10.1016/j.biomaterials.2007.02.003] [PMID: 17321590]

[409]   Bae SE, Choi J, Joung YK, Park K, Han DK. Controlled release of bone morphogenetic protein (BMP)-2 from nanocomplex incorporated on hydroxyapatite-formed titanium surface. J Control Release 2012; 160(3): 676-84.[http://dx.doi.org/10.1016/j.jconrel.2012.04.021] [PMID: 22543042]

[410]   Yoo D, Tovar N, Jimbo R, *et al.* Increased osseointegration effect of bone morphogenetic protein 2 on dental implants: an *in vivo* study. J Biomed Mater Res A 2014; 102(6): 1921-1927 .[http://dx.doi.org/10.1002/jbm.a.34862] [PMID: 23853058]

[411]   Huang YC, Kaigler D, Rice KG, Krebsbach PH, Mooney DJ. Combined angiogenic and osteogenic factor delivery enhances bone marrow stromal cell-driven bone regeneration. J Bone Miner Res 2005; 20(5): 848-57.[http://dx.doi.org/10.1359/JBMR.041226] [PMID: 15824858]

[412]   Ramazanoglu M, Lutz R, Ergun C, von Wilmowsky C, Nkenke E, Schlegel KA. The effect of combined delivery of recombinant human bone morphogenetic protein-2 and recombinant human vascular endothelial growth factor 165 from biomimetic calcium-phosphate-coated implants on osseointegration. Clin Oral Implants Res 2011; 22(12): 1433-1439 .[http://dx.doi.org/10.1111/j.1600-0501.2010.02133.x] [PMID: 21418332]

[413]   Roessler S, Born R, Scharnweber D, Worch H, Sewing A, Dard M. Biomimetic coatings functionalized with adhesion peptides for dental implants. J Mater Sci Mater Med 2001; 12(10-12): 871-7.[http://dx.doi.org/10.1023/A:1012807621414] [PMID: 15348332]

[414]   Itoh D, Yoneda S, Kuroda S, *et al.* Enhancement of osteogenesis on hydroxyapatite surface coated with synthetic peptide (EEEEEEEPRGDT) *in vitro* . J Biomed Mater Res 2002; 62(2): 292-8.[http://dx.doi.org/10.1002/jbm.10338] [PMID: 12209950]

[415]   Lutz R, Srour S, Nonhoff J, Weisel T, Damien CJ, Schlegel KA. Biofunctionalization of titanium implants with a biomimetic active peptide (P-15) promotes early osseointegration. Clin Oral Implants Res 2010; 21(7): 726-34.[http://dx.doi.org/10.1111/j.1600-0501.2009.01904.x] [PMID: 20636727]

[416]   Coelho PG, Teixeira HS, Marin C, *et al.* The *in vivo* effect of P-15 coating on early osseointegration. J Biomed Mater Res B Appl Biomater 2014; 102(3): 430-40.[http://dx.doi.org/10.1002/jbm.b.33020] [PMID: 24106136]

[417]   Ruoslahti E. RGD and other recognition sequences for integrins. Annu Rev Cell Dev Biol 1996; 12: 697-715.[http://dx.doi.org/10.1146/annurev.cellbio.12.1.697] [PMID: 8970741]

[418]   Schliephake H, Scharnweber D, Dard M, *et al.* Effect of RGD peptide coating of titanium implants on periimplant bone formation in the alveolar crest. An experimental pilot study in dogs. Clin Oral Implants Res 2002; 13(3): 312-9.[http://dx.doi.org/10.1034/j.1600-0501.2002.130312.x] [PMID: 12010163]

[419]   Elmengaard B, Bechtold JE, Søballe K. *In vivo* study of the effect of RGD treatment on bone ongrowth on press-fit titanium alloy implants. Biomaterials 2005; 26(17): 3521-3526 .[http://dx.doi.org/10.1016/j.biomaterials.2004.09.039] [PMID: 15621242]

[420]   Hennessy KM, Clem WC, Phipps MC, Sawyer AA, Shaikh FM, Bellis SL. The effect of RGD peptides on osseointegration of hydroxyapatite biomaterials. Biomaterials 2008; 29(21): 3075-3083 .[http://dx.doi.org/10.1016/j.biomaterials.2008.04.014] [PMID: 18440064]

[421]   Petrie TA, Raynor JE, Reyes CD, Burns KL, Collard DM, García AJ. The effect of integrin-specific bioactive coatings on tissue healing and implant osseointegration. Biomaterials 2008; 29(19): 2849-57.[http://dx.doi.org/10.1016/j.biomaterials.2008.03.036] [PMID: 18406458]

[422]   Dettin M, Conconi MT, Gambaretto R, *et al.* Effect of synthetic peptides on osteoblast adhesion. Biomaterials 2005; 26(22): 4507-15.[http://dx.doi.org/10.1016/j.biomaterials.2004.11.023] [PMID: 15722119]

[423] Bhatnagar RS, Qian JJ, Gough CA. The role in cell binding of a beta-bend within the triple helical region in collagen alpha 1 (I) chain: structural and biological evidence for conformational tautomerism on fiber surface. J Biomol Struct Dyn 1997; 14(5): 547-560 .[http://dx.doi.org/10.1080/07391102.1997.10508155] [PMID: 9130077]

[424] Xu T, Zhang N, Nichols HL, Shi D, Wen X. Modification of nanostructured materials for biomedical applications. Mater Sci Eng C 2007; 27: 579-94.[http://dx.doi.org/10.1016/j.msec.2006.05.029]

[425] Choi AH, Ben-Nissan B. Calcium phosphate nanocoatings and nanocomposites, part I: recent developments and advancements in tissue engineering and bioimaging. Nanomedicine (Lond) 2015; 10(14): 2249-61.[http://dx.doi.org/10.2217/nnm.15.57] [PMID: 26119630]

[426] Ben-Nissan B, Macha I, Cazalbou S, Choi AH. Calcium phosphate nanocoatings and nanocomposites, part 2: thin films for slow drug delivery and osteomyelitis. Nanomedicine (Lond) 2016; 11(5): 531-44.[http://dx.doi.org/10.2217/nnm.15.220] [PMID: 26891748]

[427] Paul W, Sharma CP. Fatty acid conjugated calcium phosphate nanoparticles for protein delivery. Int J Appl Ceram Technol 2010; 7: 129-38.[http://dx.doi.org/10.1111/j.1744-7402.2009.02442.x]

[428] Aviv M, Berdicevsky I, Zilberman M. Gentamicin-loaded bioresorbable films for prevention of bacterial infections associated with orthopedic implants. J Biomed Mater Res A 2007; 83(1): 10-9.[http://dx.doi.org/10.1002/jbm.a.31184] [PMID: 17340599]

[429] LeGeros RZ. Calcium phosphate-based osteoinductive materials. Chem Rev 2008; 108(11): 4742-53.[http://dx.doi.org/10.1021/cr800427g] [PMID: 19006399]

[430] An YH, Friedman RJ. Concise review of mechanisms of bacterial adhesion to biomaterial surfaces. J Biomed Mater Res 1998; 43(3): 338-348 .[http://dx.doi.org/10.1002/(SICI)1097-4636(199823)43:3<338::AID-JBM16>3.0.CO;2-B] [PMID: 9730073]

[431] Macha IJ, Ben-Nissan B, Milthorpe B. Improvement of elongation in nanosurface modified bioglass/PLA thin film composites. Curr Nanosci 2014; 10: 200-204 .[http://dx.doi.org/10.2174/15734137096661311290000643]

[432] Macha IJ, Cazalbou S, Ben-Nissan B, Harvey KL, Milthorpe B. Marine structure derived calcium phosphate-polymer biocomposites for local antibiotic delivery. Mar Drugs 2015; 13(1): 666-680 .[http://dx.doi.org/10.3390/md13010666] [PMID: 25608725]

[433] Macha IJ, Cazalbou S, Shimmon R, Ben-Nissan B, Milthorpe B. Development and dissolution studies of bisphosphonate (clodronate)-containing hydroxyapatite-polylactic acid biocomposites for slow drug delivery. J Tissue Eng Regen Med 2017; 11(6): 1723-31.[http://dx.doi.org/10.1002/term.2066] [PMID: 26174121]

[434] Stewart PS. Mechanisms of antibiotic resistance in bacterial biofilms. Int J Med Microbiol 2002; 292(2): 107-13.[http://dx.doi.org/10.1078/1438-4221-00196] [PMID: 12195733]

[435] Dufrêne YF. Understanding forces in biofilms. Nanomedicine (Lond) 2015; 10(8): 1219-21.[http://dx.doi.org/10.2217/nnm.15.15] [PMID: 25955121]

[436] Høiby N, Bjarnsholt T, Givskov M, Molin S, Ciofu O. Antibiotic resistance of bacterial biofilms. Int J Antimicrob Agents 2010; 35(4): 322-32.[http://dx.doi.org/10.1016/j.ijantimicag.2009.12.011] [PMID: 20149602]

[437] Mah TF, Pitts B, Pellock B, Walker GC, Stewart PS, O'Toole GA. A genetic basis for Pseudomonas aeruginosa biofilm antibiotic resistance. Nature 2003; 426(6964): 306-310 .[http://dx.doi.org/10.1038/nature02122] [PMID: 14628055]

[438] William D, Callister J. Materials science and engineering, 3rd edition. New York, John Wiley and Sons, 1994.

[439] Kendall K. Molecular adhesion and its applications. New York, Kluwer Academic/Plenum Publishers, 2001.

[440] Choi AH, Ben-Nissan B, Bendavid A, Latella B. Mechanical behavior and properties of thin films for biomedical applications.Thin Film Coatings for Materials and Biomedical Applications 2016; 117-41.[http://dx.doi.org/10.1016/B978-1-78242-453-6.00006-7]

[441] Lee LH. Fundamentals of adhesion 1991.[http://dx.doi.org/10.1007/978-1-4899-2073-7]

[442] Lawn BR. Fracture of brittle solids 1993.[http://dx.doi.org/10.1017/CBO9780511623127]

[443] Lane M. Interface fracture. Annu Rev Mater Res 2003; 33: 29-54 .[http://dx.doi.org/10.1146/annurev.matsci.33.012202.130440]

[444] Aladjem A. Anodic oxidation of titanium and its alloys. J Mater Sci 1973; 8: 688-704.[http://dx.doi.org/10.1007/BF00561225]

[445] Andreeva V, Shishakov N. Z Fis Khim 1958; 32: 1671

[446] Andreeva V, Kazarin V. Proc III Internat Conf Met Corrosion 1969; 1966

[447] Schutz RW, Thomas DE. ASM Metals Handbook of Corrosion, Vol 13 UK, ASM International, 1987

[448] Davis JR. Metals Handbook Desk Edition. 2nd edition, Ohio, ASM International, 1998.

[449] Brunette DM, Tengvall P, Textor M, Thomsen P. Titanium in medicine: materials science, surface science, engineering, biological responses and medical applications (engineering materials) Heidelburg, Springer, 2001 [http://dx.doi.org/10.1007/978-3-642-56486-4]

[450] Tomashov N, Strukov N. Dakl Akad Nauk SSSR 1963; 152: 1177

[451] Kossyi G, Nivakoyskii V, Kolotyrkin YA. Zashchita Metallov 1969; 5: 210

[452] Arsov LD. Growth of anodic oxide films on titanium surfaces, in: Contemporary inorganic materials: process in ceramics, metals and composites, 7th German-Yugoslav meeting on engineering materials science and technology, Bad Herranalb, Kernforschungsanlage, Julich 1985.

[453] Guntherschnise A, Betz H. Z Phys 1934; 92: 367 [http://dx.doi.org/10.1007/BF01340820]

[454] Nakata N, Iida Y. Denki Kagaku Oyobi Kogyo Bulsuri Kagaku 1969; 37: 366

[455] Hall C, Hackerman N. Charging processes on anodic polarization of titanium. J Phys Chem 1953; 57: 262-8.[http://dx.doi.org/10.1021/j150504a002]

[456] Kover F, Musselin M. A comparative study of anodic oxide films on titanium, niobium and tantalum. Thin Solid Films 1968; 2: 211-34.[http://dx.doi.org/10.1016/0040-6090(68)90003-5]

[457] Krasilśhchikov A. Proc III Inter Conf Met Corrosion 1968; 1966

[458] Tylecote R. CNRS Symp 1963; 122

[459] Dornelas W. Thesis, University of Paris, France, 1967

[460] Cheseldine DM. Anodic oxidation of titanium in formic acid electrolytes. J Electrochem Soc 1964; 111: 1005-7.[http://dx.doi.org/10.1149/1.2426282]

[461] Bogoyavlenskii A. Tr Kaz Aviats Inst 1966; 90: 3

[462] Tomashov I, Matveeva T. Zashchita Metallov 1971; 7: 272

[463] Cotton JB. Proc III Internat Conf Met Corrosion 1969; 1966

[464] Lepienski CM, Pharr GM, Park YJ, Watkins TR, Misra A, Zhang X. Factors limiting the measurement of residual stresses in thin films by nanoindentation. Thin Solid Films 2004; 447: 215-57.

[465] Stoney GG. The tension of metallic films deposited by electrolysis. Proc R Soc Lond 1909; 82: 172-5.[http://dx.doi.org/10.1098/rspa.1909.0021]

[466] Tsui YC, Doyle C, Clyne TW. Plasma sprayed hydroxyapatite coatings on titanium substrates. Part 1: Mechanical properties and residual stress levels. Biomaterials 1998; 19(22): 2015-2029 .[http://dx.doi.org/10.1016/S0142-9612(98)00103-3] [PMID: 9870753]

[467] Nix DW. Mechanical properties of thin films (class notes for a graduate class at Stanford University), iMechanica, 2006.

[468] Mittal KL. Adhesion measurement of films and coatings: A commentary. In: Mittal KL, Ed. Adhesion measurements of films and coatings. Utrecht, VSP, 1995. Adhesion measurements of films and coatings 1995.

[469] Benjamin P, Weaver C. Measurement of adhesion of thin films. Proc R Soc Lond A Math Phys Sci 1960; 254: 163-76.[http://dx.doi.org/10.1098/rspa.1960.0012]

[470] Laugier MT. The development of the scratch test technique for the determination of the adhesion of coatings. Thin Solid Films 1981; 76: 289-94.[http://dx.doi.org/10.1016/0040-6090(81)90700-8]

[471] Laugier MT. An energy approach to the adhesion of coatings using the scratch test. Thin Solid Films 1984; 117: 243-9.[http://dx.doi.org/10.1016/0040-6090(84)90354-7]

[472] Burnett PJ, Rickerby DS. The relationship between hardness and scratch adhesion. Thin Solid Films 1987; 154: 403-16.[http://dx.doi.org/10.1016/0040-6090(87)90382-8]

[473] Bull S, Berasetegui E. An overview of the potential of quantitative coating adhesion measurement by scratch testing. Tribol Int 2009; 39: 99-114.[http://dx.doi.org/10.1016/j.triboint.2005.04.013]

[474] Burnett PJ, Rickerby DS. The scratch adhesion test: an elastic-plastic indentation analysis. Thin Solid Films 1988; 157: 233-54.[http://dx.doi.org/10.1016/0040-6090(88)90006-5]

[475] Bull SJ, Rickerby DS, Matthews A, Leyland A, Pace AR, Valli J. The use of scratch adhesion testing for the determination of interfacial adhesion - the importance of frictional drag. Surf Coat Tech 1988; 36: 503-17.[http://dx.doi.org/10.1016/0257-8972(88)90178-8]

[476] Hutchinson JW, Suo Z. Mixed-mode cracking in layered structures. Adv Appl Mech 1991; 29: 64.[http://dx.doi.org/10.1016/S0065-2156(08)70164-9]

[477] Venkataraman SK, Kohlstedt DL, Gerberich WW. Metal ceramic interfacial fracture-resistance using the continuous microscratch technique. Thin Solid Films 1993; 223: 269-275 .[http://dx.doi.org/10.1016/0040-6090(93)90532-T]

[478] Cheng K, Ren CB, Weng WJ, *et al.* Bonding strength of fluoridated hydroxyapatite coatings: a comparative study on pull-out and scratch analysis. Thin Solid Films 2009; 517: 5361-5364 .[http://dx.doi.org/10.1016/j.tsf.2009.03.122]

[479] Wei M, Ruys AJ, Swain MV, Kim SH, Milthorpe BK, Sorrell CC. Interfacial bond strength of electrophoretically deposited hydroxyapatite coatings on metals. J Mater Sci Mater Med 1999; 10(7): 401-9.[http://dx.doi.org/10.1023/A:1008923029945] [PMID: 15348125]

[480] Bennett SJ, Devries KL, Williams ML. Adhesive fracture mechanics. Int J Fract 1974; 10: 33-43.[http://dx.doi.org/10.1007/BF00955077]

[481] Agrawal DC, Raj R. Measurement of the ultimate shear-strength of a metal ceramic interface. Acta Metall 1989; 37: 1265-70.[http://dx.doi.org/10.1016/0001-6160(89)90120-X]

[482] Agrawal DC, Raj R. Ultimate shear strengths of copper silica and nickel silica interfaces. Mater Sci Eng A 1990; 126: 125-31.[http://dx.doi.org/10.1016/0921-5093(90)90118-M]

[483] Ignat M. Mechanical response of multilayers submitted to *in-situ* experiments. Key Eng Mater 1996; 116-117: 279-90.[http://dx.doi.org/10.4028/www.scientific.net/KEM.116-117.279]

[484] Latella BA, Triani G, Zhang Z, Short KT, Bartlett JR, Ignat M. Enhanced adhesion of atomic layer deposited titania on polycarbonate substrates. Thin Solid Films 2007; 515: 3138-45.[http://dx.doi.org/10.1016/j.tsf.2006.08.022]

[485] Ignat M, Marieb T, Fukimoto H, Flinn PA. Mechanical behaviour of submicron multilayers submitted to microtensile experiments. Thin Solid Films 1999; 353: 201-207 .[http://dx.doi.org/10.1016/S0040-6090(99)00397-1]

[486] Latella BA, Ignat M, Barbé CJ, Cassidy DJ, Li H. Cracking and decohesion of sol-gel hybrid coatings on metallic substrates. J Sol-Gel Sci Technol 2004; 31: 143-149 .[http://dx.doi.org/10.1023/B:JSST.0000047976.41395.51]

[487] Latella BA, Gan BK, Davies KE, Mckenzie DR, Mcculloch DG. Titanium nitride/vanadium nitride alloy coatings: mechanical properties and adhesion characteristics. Surf Coat Tech 2006; 200: 3605-11.[http://dx.doi.org/10.1016/j.surfcoat.2004.09.008]

[488] Beuth JL, Klingbeil NW. Cracking of thin films bonded to elastic-plastic substrates. J Mech Phys Solids 1996; 44: 1411-28.[http://dx.doi.org/10.1016/0022-5096(96)00042-7]

[489] Latella BA, Ignat M. Interface fracture surface energy of sol-gel bonded silicon wafers by three-point bending. J Mater Sci Mater Electron 2012; 23: 8-13.[http://dx.doi.org/10.1007/s10854-011-0381-2]

[490] Charalambides PG, Lund J, Evans AG, McMeeking RM. A test specimen for determining the fracture resistance of bimaterial interfaces. J Appl Mech 1989; 56: 77-82.[http://dx.doi.org/10.1115/1.3176069]

[491] Saha R, Nix WD. Effects of the substrate on the determination of thin film mechanical properties by nanoindentation. Acta Mater 2002; 50: 23-38.[http://dx.doi.org/10.1016/S1359-6454(01)00328-7]

[492] Field JS, Swain MV. Determining the mechanical properties of small volumes of material from submicrometer spherical indentations. J Mater Res 1995; 10: 101-112 .[http://dx.doi.org/10.1557/JMR.1995.0101]

[493] Field JS, Swain MV. A simple predictive model for spherical indentation. J Mater Res 1993; 8: 297-306.[http://dx.doi.org/10.1557/JMR.1993.0297]

[494] Fischer-Cripps AC. Introduction to nanoindentation. New York, Springer, 2002. [http://dx.doi.org/10.1007/978-0-387-22462-6]

[495] Liu P, Zhang YW, Zeng KY, Lu C, Lam KY. Finite element analysis of interface delamination and buckling in thin film systems by wedge indentation. Eng Fract Mech 2007; 74: 1118-1125 .[http://dx.doi.org/10.1016/j.engfracmech.2006.12.025]

[496] Sauer RA, Mergel JC. A geometrically exact finite beam element formulation for thin film adhesion and debonding. Finite Elem Anal Des 2014; 86: 120-35.[http://dx.doi.org/10.1016/j.finel.2014.03.009]

[497] Sun Z, Wan KT, Dillard DA. A theoretical and numerical study of thin film delamination using the pull-off test. Int J Solids Struct 2004; 41: 717-30.[http://dx.doi.org/10.1016/j.ijsolstr.2003.09.027]

[498] Sun Z, Dillard DA. Three-dimensional finite element analysis of fracture modes for the pull-off test of a thin film from a stiff substrate. Thin Solid Films 2010; 518: 3837-3843 .[http://dx.doi.org/10.1016/j.tsf.2009.11.008]

SUBJECT INDEX

www.ingramcontent.com/pod-product-compliance
Lightning Source LLC
Chambersburg PA
CBHW050839220326
41598CB00006B/408